A
Handbook
of
Routine
Urinalysis

Sister Laurine Graff

MS, CLS, MT(ASCP)

A Handbook of Routine Urinalysis

J. B. Lippincott Company

Philadelphia   London   Mexico City   New York
St. Louis   São Paulo   Sydney

Acquisitions Editor: Lisa A. Biello
Sponsoring Editor: Sanford J. Robinson
Manuscript Editor: Randi Boyette
Indexer: Julia B. Schwager
Art Director: Maria S. Karkucinski

Designer: Patrick Turner
Production Supervisor: N. Carol Kerr
Production Assistant: J. Corey Gray
Compositor: Progressive Typographers
Printer/Binder: Kingsport Press

3 5 6 4 2

Library of Congress Cataloging in Publication Data

Graff, Laurine.
    A handbook of routine urinalysis.

    Revision of thesis (M.S.)—San Francisco State
University.
    Bibliography.
    Includes index.
    1. Urine—Analysis—Handbooks, manuals, etc.
    2. Urine—Examination—Handbooks, manuals, etc.
    I. Title.   [DNLM: 1. Urine—Analysis—Handbooks.
QY 185 G736h]
RB53.G73   1982   616.07′566   82-15174
ISBN 0-397-52111-1   AACR2

The term "routine urinalysis" describes a series of screening tests that are capable of detecting a variety of renal, urinary tract, and systemic diseases.

The purpose of this text is to provide a handbook of routine urinalysis that can serve as an instructional aid for medical technology students and other laboratory personnel, and also as a reference book in the medical laboratory. *A Handbook of Routine Urinalysis* presents a simple clinical explanation of the various properties and constituents of urine that are tested in the routine urinalysis. It discusses the principles of the tests, provides an explanation of abnormal results, and gives several procedures that can be used as alternative or confirmatory tests. By means of 231 color photomicrographs, the book attempts to familiarize the student or reader with both the normal and abnormal structures found in the urinary sediment.

Chapter 5 contains some special screening procedures that are not part of the routine urinalysis. Some of these procedures can be used for confirmatory testing, while the others, because of their qualitative nature, are usually relegated to the routine urinalysis personnel.

The information in Chapter 2 concerning the reactions of the various dipstick tests was up-to-date at the time the book was written. Since the manufacturers frequently try to improve their products, the reagents, sensitivities, detection ranges, and timings may change. It is, therefore, important to follow the manufacturer's most recent directions and use a current color chart.

For the benefit of any individual who may wish to take photomicrographs of urinary sediment, I would like to share a few discoveries that I made, at the expense of several rolls of film and many good specimens. I found that the type of slide film that is meant for use with tungsten light resulted in pictures that were bluish-gray in color. You may notice some of these in the book. When I used daylight film with the appropriate blue filter as mentioned in the manufacturer's directions (which was supposed to compensate for the tungsten light source), the result was blue photos. I found that I got the best results, with true color, by using daylight film without any filters.

I would also like to mention that with only two exceptions, the photomicrographs in this book are of unstained urinary sediment, so the color that you see is the color of the structure itself.

Sister Laurine Graff
MS, CLS, MT(ASCP)

Acknowledgments

I would like to again thank those individuals who helped in the original formulation of this book as a Master's thesis at San Francisco State University. In addition, I would like to thank: Marie Luciani, Managing Editor of Medcom, Inc., and Dr. George Schreiner for the use of Figures 3-24 and 3-28; Dr. Kenneth A. Borchardt for the use of Figure 3-73; Dr. Gregory Antipa of San Francisco State University and Dr. John R. Krause of the University of Pittsburgh for the use of their photomicroscopes; and Lisa A. Biello of the J.B. Lippincott Company for her encouragement and assistance.

In a special way, I wish to express my appreciation to my religious community, the Sisters of Divine Providence, for supporting me in this project.

Contents

List of Figures   *xiii*

1   An Introduction to Urinalysis   **1**

The Formation of Urine   2
Collection of Specimen   7
  Methods   7
  Preservation   8
  Timing   9
Examination of Physical Characteristics   10
  Character   10
    Color   10
    Appearance   13
  Specific Gravity   13
    Urinometer   15
    Refractometer   16
    Specific Gravity Reagent Strips   18
    Specific Gravity vs. Osmolality   18

2   Chemical Examination   **21**

Urinary pH   23
  Reagent Test-Strips   26
Protein   26
  Screening Tests   29
    Reagent Test-Strips   29
    Sulfosalicylic Acid   31
    Heat and Acetic Acid Test   32
    Heller's Ring Test   32
  Bence-Jones Protein   33
    Heat Precipitation Test   35
    Toluene Sulfonic Acid Test   35
Glucose and Other Reducing Substances   36
  Glucose Oxidase Test   38
  Screening for Reducing Substances   40
    Clinitest Tablets   40
    Benedict's Qualitative Test   42
Ketones   43
  Reagent Test-Strips   45
  Acetest Tablets   46
  Rothera's Test   46

Gerhardt's Test   47
Hart's Test   48
Occult Blood   48
Hematuria   49
Hemoglobinuria   50
Myoglobinuria   52
Screening Tests   52
Reagent Test-Strips   53
Hematest   54
Ammonium Sulfate Test   55
Bilirubin and Urobilinogen   55
Screening Tests for Bilirubin (Bile)   59
Reagent Test-Strips   59
Ictotest   60
Foam Test   60
Smith Iodine Test   61
Harrison Spot Test   61
Screening Tests for Urobilinogen   61
Reagent Test-Strips   62
Ehrlich's Qualitative Test   63
Nitrite   64
N-Multistix   64
Chemstrip 8   65
Quality Control and Instrumentation   65

**3   Microscopic Examination of the
Urinary Sediment**   **69**

Preparation of the Sediment and Use of the Microscope   72
Cells   74
Erythrocytes   74
Leukocytes   77
Epithelial Cells   79
Renal Tubular Epithelial Cells   80
Transitional Epithelial Cells   81
Squamous Epithelial Cells   81
Crystals   83
Acid Urine   83
Uric Acid Crystals   83
Calcium Oxalate Crystals   89
Amorphous Urates   90
Hippuric Acid Crystals   90
Sodium Urates   90
Calcium Sulfate Crystals   92
Cystine Crystals   92
Leucine   94
Tyrosine   94

Cholesterol   96
Sulfa and Other Drug Crystals   97
Alkaline Urine   101
Triple Phosphates   102
Amorphous Phosphates   102
Calcium Carbonate   103
Calcium Phosphate   103
Ammonium Biurates   105
Casts   107
Hyaline Casts   108
Red Cell Casts   108
White Cell Casts   109
Granular Casts   111
Epithelial Cell Casts   111
Waxy Casts   111
Fatty Casts   115
Miscellaneous Structures   116
Bacteria   116
Yeast   117
Cylindroids   117
Spermatozoa   118
Mucous Threads   118
Oval Fat Bodies and Free Fat Droplets   120
Artifacts   122
Starch Crystals   122
Fibers   124
Oil Droplets   125
Miscellaneous Structures   125
Parasites   129

4   An Atlas of Urinary Sediment   **133**

5   Special Screening Procedures   **241**

Ascorbic Acid   242
C-Stix   242
Stix   242
Rous Test for Hemosiderin (Prussian Blue Reaction)   243
Reagent Test-Strip for Leukocytes   243
Lignin Test for Sulfonamides   244
Homogentisic Acid   245
Ferric Chloride Test   245
Alkali Test   246
Film Test   246
Melanin   246
Ferric Chloride Test   246
Bromine Test   246

Thormählen Test for Melanogen   247
Phenylketonuria   247
  Phenistix   249
  Ferric Chloride Test   250
Inborn Errors of Metabolism   250
  Aminoaciduria   251
  Screening Tests   252
    Ferric Chloride Test   254
    Cetyltrimethylammonium Bromide Test   255
    Dinitrophenylhydrazine Test   256
    Cyanide–Nitroprusside Test   257
    Nitrosonaphthol Test   258
    Ninhydrin Test   259
Porphyrins and Porphobilinogen   259
  Porphyrin Screening Test   261
  Watson-Schwartz Test   262
  Hoesch Test for Porphobilinogen   264

Bibliography   *265*

Index   *275*

List of Figures

1-1. The urinary tract 3
1-2. The kidney and nephron 4
1-3. Urinometer for measuring specific gravity 15
1-4. Schematic diagram of the Total Solids Refractometer 17
2-1. *A.* Normal pathway of bilirubin and urobilinogen 56
    B. Pathway in hepatic jaundice 57
    C. Pathway in obstructive jaundice 58
    D. Pathway in hemolytic jaundice 58
3-1. Amorphous phosphates and hyaline cylindroid 73
3-2. Red blood cells 75
3-3. RBCs and WBCs 76
3-4. White blood cells in a hypotonic urine 77
3-5. White cell clumps 78
3-6. Numerous white cells 79
3-7. Renal epithelial cells and numerous white cells 80
3-8. Transitional epithelial cells 81
3-9. Transitional epithelial cell, several squamous epithelial cells and white cells 82
3-10. Squamous epithelial cells 82
3-11. Crystals frequently found in acid urine 85
3-12. Other crystals found in acid urine 86
3-13. Uric acid crystals 87
3-14. Uric acid crystals in rosette formation 87
3-15. Six-sided uric acid crystal 88
3-16. Polarized uric acid crystal 88
3-17. Calcium oxalate crystal 89
3-18. Calcium oxalate crystals and squamous epithelial cells 90
3-19. Amorphous urates 91
3-20. Hippuric acid crystal 91
3-21. Sodium urate crystals 92
3-22. Cystine crystal 93
3-23. Cystine crystals 93
3-24. Leucine spheroids and WBCs 94
3-25. Tyrosine crystals 95

3-26. Same tyrosine crystals as Figure 3-25, but under a higher power 95

3-27. Cholesterol crystal with typical notched edges 96

3-28. Sulfonamide crystals 97

3-29. X-ray dye crystals (Hypaque) 98

3-30. X-ray dye crystals (Renografin) 99

3-31. X-ray dye crystals (Hypaque) 99

3-32. Polarized x-ray dye crystals 100

3-33. Bilirubin crystals 100

3-34. Crystals found in alkaline urine 101

3-35. Triple phosphate crystals 102

3-36. Amorphous phosphates 103

3-37. Calcium carbonate crystals 104

3-38. Calcium phosphate crystals 104

3-39. Calcium phosphate plate or phosphate sheath 105

3-40. Ammonium biurate crystals 106

3-41. Ammonium biurate crystals without spicules 106

3-42. Hyaline cast and red blood cells 109

3-43. Red cell cast and RBCs 110

3-44. White cell cast and WBCs 110

3-45. Finely granular casts 112

3-46. Broad coarsely granular cast 112

3-47. Epithelial cell cast 113

3-48. Waxy cast and WBCs 114

3-49. Waxy cast, WBCs, and bacteria 114

3-50. Fatty cast 115

3-51. Bacteria (rods, cocci, and chains) 116

3-52. Yeast cells 117

3-53. Cylindroid 118

3-54. Spermatozoa 119

3-55. Mucous threads 119

3-56. Oval fat body and a fiber 121

3-57. Fat droplets 121

3-58. Polarized anisotropic fat droplets 122

3-59. Starch crystal 123

3-60. Polarized starch crystals 123

3-61. Cloth fibers 124

3-62. Fibers 125

3-63. Fiber 126

3-64. Oil droplet 126

3-65. Hair and a coarsely granular cast 127

3-66. Glass fragments   127

3-67. Air bubble and amorphous urates   128

3-68. Talcum powder particles   128

3-69. Fecal contamination   129

3-70. *Trichomonas vaginalis*   130

3-71. *Enterobius vermicularis* ovum and WBCs   130

3-72. Head of the *Enterobius vermicularis* adult female worm   131

3-73. *Schistosoma haematobium* ovum   132

4-1. Hypotonic urine containing WBCs, 1 RBC, 2 renal epithelial cells, and a transitional epithelial cell   134

4-2. Epithelial cells, WBCs, RBCs, and bacteria   134

4-3. Many RBCs and a squamous epithelial cell   135

4-4. White cells, a few red cells, and bacteria   136

4-5. Large clump of WBCs and many squamous epithelial cells   136

4-6. Distorted white cells   137

4-7. Clump of WBCs and 4 epithelial cells, all of which have been stained with bilirubin   138

4-8. White cells and squamous epithelial cells   138

4-9. Renal epithelial cells   139

4-10. Sheet of squamous epithelial cells and WBCs   140

4-11. Numerous white cells and a few transitional epithelial cells   140

4-12. Squamous epithelial cells and calcium oxalates   141

4-13. Amorphous urates   142

4-14. Amorphous urates   142

4-15. Uric acid crystals, diamond or rhombic form   143

4-16. Uric acid crystals in the urine of a patient with a kidney stone   144

4-17. White cell cast, finely granular cast, and uric acid crystals   144

4-18. Uric acid crystals in rosette formation   145

4-19. Atypical form of uric acid crystals   146

4-20. Formation of uric acid crystals   146

4-21. Thick rosette formations of uric acid crystals under low power magnification   147

4-22. Thick rosette formation under a higher power magnification   148

4-23. Uric acid crystals and calcium oxalates   148

4-24. Polarized uric acid crystals   149

4-25. Polarized uric acid crystal   150

4-26. Uric acid crystals in a pseudocast formation   150

4-27. Calcium oxalate crystals   151

4-28. Calcium oxalate crystals   152

4-29. Calcium oxalates, amorphous urates, and a piece of debris   152

4-30. Calcium oxalate crystals clustered around a piece of debris   153

4-31. Calcium oxalates and amorphous urates   154

4-32. Hippuric acid crystals   154

4-33. Sodium urate crystals   155

4-34. Sodium urates and a WBC   156

4-35. Sodium urate crystals   156

4-36. Cystine crystals   157

4-37. Cystine crystal with unequal sides   158

4-38. Cystine crystals and WBCs   158

4-39. Cystine crystal with a layered or laminated surface   159

4-40. Cystine crystals, few WBCs, and squamous epithelial cells   160

4-41. Cystine crystals and a squamous epithelial cell   160

4-42. Cystine crystals   161

4-43. Cystine crystals of various sizes   162

4-44. Cystine crystal with a pitted surface   162

4-45. Cystine crystals in a pseudocast formation   163

4-46. Tyrosine crystals   164

4-47. Tyrosine crystals   164

4-48. Tyrosine crystals   165

4-49. Tyrosine crystals   166

4-50. Tyrosine crystals   166

4-51. X-ray dye crystals   167

4-52. X-ray dye crystals   168

4-53. Polarized x-ray dye crystals   168

4-54. Bilirubin crystals and bilirubin-stained WBCs and granular cast   169

4-55. Bilirubin crystals, fat droplets, and bilirubin-stained sediment   170

4-56. Triple phosphate crystals   170

4-57. Triple phosphates and amorphous phosphates   171

4-58. Triple phosphate crystals   172

4-59. Triple phosphate crystals   172

4-60. Triple phosphate crystals and amorphous phosphates   173

4-61. Triple phosphate crystals   174

4-62. Triple phosphate crystals 174

4-63. Triple phosphate crystal and mucous 175

4-64. Triple phosphate crystal 176

4-65. Calcium phosphate crystals 176

4-66. Calcium phosphate plates and amorphous phosphates 177

4-67. Calcium phosphate plate (or phosphate sheath) and amorphous phosphates 178

4-68. Ammonium biurate crystals 178

4-69. Ammonium biurates 179

4-70. Ammonium biurate crystals 180

4-71. Ammonium biurates, mucous, and a WBC 180

4-72. Ammonium biurate crystals 181

4-73. Ammonium biurate crystal and a squamous epithelial cell 182

4-74. Ammonium biurates 182

4-75. Ammonium biurates without spicules 183

4-76. Ammonium biurate crystals, spheroid form 184

4-77. Hyaline cast, WBCs, 4 RBCs, and bacteria 184

4-78. Hyaline casts 185

4-79. Hyaline cast that is bent back upon itself, and many RBCs 186

4-80. Hyaline casts and many RBCs 186

4-81. Hyaline casts 187

4-82. Hyaline cast 188

4-83. Many hyaline and WBC casts, and rare red blood cell 188

4-84. Hyaline cast, WBCs, RBCs, and epithelial cells 189

4-85. Hyaline cast with a few granular inclusions 190

4-86. Convoluted red cell cast 190

4-87. Red cell cast and many RBCs 191

4-88. Red cell cast 192

4-89. Red cell cast 192

4-90. Red cell cast and amorphous urates 193

4-91. White cell cast, WBCs, squamous epithelial cells, and mucous 194

4-92. White cell cast 194

4-93. White cell cast 195

4-94. Bilirubin-stained casts, fibers, and sediment 196

4-95. Mixed cast, WBCs, RBCs, and rare epithelial cell 196

4-96. Bilirubin-stained WBC cast or granular cast? 197

4-97. Many white cell casts and many WBCs 198

4-98. Bilirubin-stained granular cast 198

4-99. Finely granular cast 199

4-100. Finely granular cast, WBCs, and bacteria 200

4-101. Broad granular cast 200

4-102. Finely granular casts, WBCs, and RBCs 201

4-103. Finely granular casts and WBCs 202

4-104. Finely granular casts and WBCs 202

4-105. Coarsely granular cast 203

4-106. Coarsely granular cast 204

4-107. Coarsely granular cast, calcium phosphate plate, and amorphous phosphates 204

4-108. Coarsely granular cast 205

4-109. Granular cast 206

4-110. Waxy cast and amorphous urates 206

4-111. Bilirubin-stained waxy cast, granular cast, WBCs, and amorphous sediment 207

4-112. Long waxy cast, WBCs, and epithelial cells 208

4-113. Finely granular cast becoming a waxy cast 208

4-114. Convoluted waxy cast 209

4-115. Convoluted waxy cast 210

4-116. Epithelial cell cast 210

4-117. Mixed cast 211

4-118. Mixed cast, yeast cells, and a WBC 212

4-119. Mixed cast 212

4-120. Many casts, WBCs, RBCs, and amorphous sediment, all of which are stained with bilirubin 213

4-121. Broad, mixed granular and RBC cast, and a broad granular cast 214

4-122. Granular cylindroid 214

4-123. Hyaline cylindroid 215

4-124. Bacteria 216

4-125. Yeast, WBCs, rare RBC, and bacteria 216

4-126. Yeast cells 217

4-127. Finely granular cast and yeast 218

4-128. Sperm and epithelial cells 218

4-129. Mucous which contains WBCs and RBCs 219

4-130. Fat droplets and epithelial cells 220

4-131. Oval fat body, granular cast, and amorphous urates 220

4-132. Oval fat body 221

4-133. Oval fat body 222

4-134. Oval fat body and WBCs 222

4-135. Oval fat body 223

4-136. Oval fat body 224

4-137. Oval fat body 224

4-138. Starch crystals and amorphous urates 225

4-139. Starch crystals 226

4-140. Polarized starch crystals showing the typical "Maltese-cross" formation 226

4-141. Debris from a diaper 227

4-142. Finely granular cast and WBCs 228

4-143. Fiber 228

4-144. Fiber 229

4-145. Fiber 230

4-146. Fiber 230

4-147. Debris from a diaper 231

4-148. Fibers 232

4-149. Fibers 232

4-150. Fiber 233

4-151. Fibers 234

4-152. Fiber, calcium oxalate crystals, and amorphous urates 234

4-153. Fiber 235

4-154. Air bubbles, phosphate plate, and amorphous phosphates 236

4-155. Talcum powder particles and a few squamous epithelial cells 236

4-156. Pinworm ovum and WBCs 237

4-157. *Enterobius vermicularis* or pinworm ovum 238

4-158. Tail of the adult female pinworm 238

4-159. Pinworm ovum and WBCs 239

5-1. The normal metabolic pathway of phenylalanine and tyrosine 245

5-2. Increased formation of phenylalanine metabolites resulting from the deficiency of phenylalanine hydroxylase 248

5-3. Biosynthesis of heme 260

1

An Introduction to Urinalysis

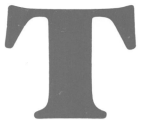he physical and chemical properties of urine have long been recognized as important indicators of health. It is the purpose of this book to present an explanation of the tests included in a routine urinalysis, and also to include some of the screening tests which are requested to be done on random urine samples.

The term "screening" implies that a positive result should be followed up by further studies such as quantitative tests. The scope of this handbook will not include these quantitative procedures.

A routine urinalysis, which is frequently referred to as an R+M (routine and microscopic), includes examination for urinary color, appearance, specific gravity, pH, protein, glucose, ketones, and occult blood, as well as a microscopic examination of the sediment. Because of the recent production of dipsticks that are capable of measuring seven or eight parameters, some laboratories now include bilirubin, nitrite, and urobilinogen in the routine urinalysis. An R+M on a young child should also include a screening test for reducing substances in order to allow for the early detection of congenital defects in carbohydrate metabolism.

In spite of all the technical advances in the clinical laboratory, the value of a urinalysis is dependent upon the ability of the technologist who performs it. Care must be taken to properly interpret and evaluate the various tests. It is the aim of this book to provide a simple explanation of these tests, and by means of photomicrographs to familiarize the reader with the structures found in the urinary sediment.

The Formation of Urine

The kidneys are paired organs which are located in the small of the back on each side of the spine. They are responsible for maintaining homeostasis including the regulation of body fluids, acid–base balance, electrolyte balance and the excretion of waste products. They are also concerned with the maintenance of blood pressure and erythropoiesis. Renal function is influenced by the blood volume, pressure, and composition, as well as by the adrenal and pituitary glands.

The formation of urine involves the complex processes of blood filtration, the reabsorption of essential substances including water, and the tubular secretion of certain substances. After formation in the kidney, the urine passes down the ureter into the bladder, where it is temporarily stored before being excreted through the urethra (Fig. 1-1).

The nephron is the functional unit of the kidney and there are approximately one million nephrons in each kidney. The nephron consists of a capillary network, called the glomerulus, and a long

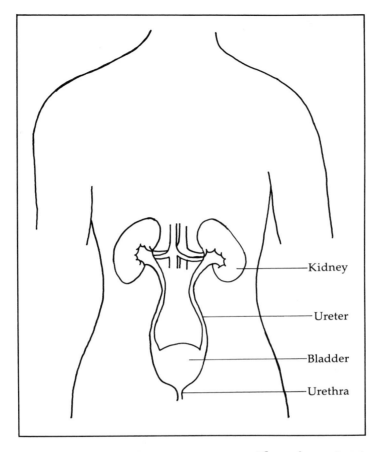

The urinary tract.   **FIGURE 1-1**

tubule which is divided into three parts: the proximal convoluted tubule, the loop of Henle, and the distal convoluted tubule. Each nephron empties into a collecting tubule to which other nephrons are connected. The urine then collects in the renal pelvis and empties into the ureter. The glomerulus and the convoluted tubules are located in the cortex of the kidney, while the loop of Henle extends down into the medulla. In Figure 1-2 the nephron has been stretched out and the surrounding blood vessels removed in order to demonstrate the different sections of the tubule.

   Approximately 20–25% of the blood that leaves the left ventricle of the heart enters the kidneys by way of the renal arteries. This means that in a normal adult the blood passes through the kidneys at a rate of about 1200 ml/min, or 600 ml/min/kidney. After the renal artery enters the kidney it breaks up into smaller branches until thousands of tiny arterioles are formed. These arterioles are called afferent arterioles because they carry the blood to the nephrons. Each afferent arteriole then forms the capillary network of a glomerulus.

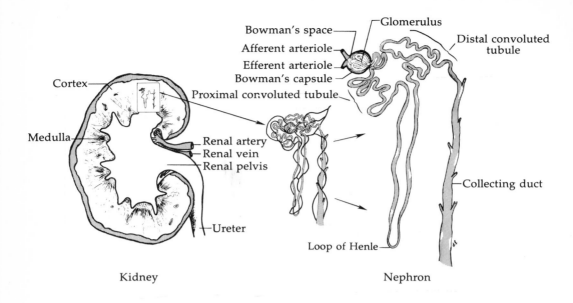

Kidney   Nephron

FIGURE 1-2   **The kidney and nephron.**

The glomerulus is surrounded by a structure called the Bowman's capsule, and the space that is formed between the capsule and the glomerulus is the Bowman's space. As a result of its special structure, the glomerular wall acts as an ultrafilter which is very permeable to water. The pressure of the blood within the glomerulus forces water and dissolved solutes with a molecular weight of less than 50,000 through the semipermeable capillary membrane and into the Bowman's space (Shaw and Benson 1974). The remainder of the blood including blood cells, plasma proteins, and large molecules, leaves the glomerulus via the efferent arteriole and enters a second capillary network, called the peritubular capillaries, which surrounds the tubules.

Approximately 120 ml/min, or one-fifth, of the renal plasma is filtered through the glomeruli forming what is known as the ultrafiltrate. The ultrafiltrate has the same composition as blood plasma but it is normally free of protein except for about 10 mg/dl of low-molecular-weight protein (Sisson 1976). Some of the filtered products include water, glucose, electrolytes, amino acids, urea, uric acid, creatinine, and ammonia.

As the glomerular filtrate passes through the proximal tubules, a large portion of the water, sodium chloride, bicarbonate, potassium, calcium, amino acids, phosphate, protein, glucose, and other threshold substances needed by the body are reabsorbed and pass back into the bloodstream. These substances are reabsorbed in varying proportions so that while proteins and glucose, for example, appear to be almost completely reabsorbed, sodium chloride is only partly reabsorbed, and there is no reabsorption of creatinine. Over 80% of the filtrate is reabsorbed in the proximal tubule. The unique structure of the proximal tubule makes this reabsorption possible. The epithelial cells that line this portion of the tubule have a brush border of microvilli which provides a large surface area for reabsorption and secretion. These microvilli contain various enzymes such as carbonic anhydrase which help in these processes (Bennett and Glassnock n.d.).

Threshold substances are those substances which are almost completely reabsorbed by the renal tubules when their concentration in the plasma is within normal limits. When the normal plasma level is exceeded, the substance is no longer totally reabsorbed and therefore appears in the urine. Glucose is a high threshold substance because it usually does not appear in the urine until the plasma concentration exceeds about 160 to 180 mg/dl. Some of the other threshold substances include sodium chloride, amino acids, potassium, creatine, and ascorbic acid.

As the filtrate moves through the tubules, various substances are added to it by the process of tubular secretion. In the proximal tubule, sulfates, glucuronides, hippurates, hydrogen ions, and drugs such as penicillin are some of the substances which are secreted. In the proximal as well as the distal tubule, the hydrogen ions are exchanged for the sodium ions of sodium bicarbonate. The hydrogen ions then combine with the bicarbonate in the filtrate to form carbonic acid which in the presence of carbonic anhydrase breaks down to water and carbon dioxide. The carbon dioxide then diffuses back out of the tubule, and thus, both the sodium and bicarbonate are reabsorbed.

Like the proximal tubule, the descending limb of the loop of Henle is very permeable to water, but the resorption of solutes does not occur in this part of the loop (Murphy and Henry 1979). The ascending limb, however, is nearly impermeable to water, but there is active resorption of sodium, chloride, calcium, and magnesium. As a result of the loss of sodium chloride, the fluid that leaves the loop of Henle has a lower osmolality than plasma. In this section of the tubule and in the remaining tubule, hydrogen ion and ammonia are secreted.

The mechanism that provides for the absorption of water from the descending loop, and the resorption of solute without water in the ascending limb, is called countercurrent multiplication. There is a set of blood vessels called the "vasa recta" that is parallel to and shaped the same as Henle's loop. In the vasa recta, solute diffuses out of the interstitium of the medulla and into the ascending limb, and then out of the ascending limb back into the interstitium. Water, however, moves in the opposite direction or out of the descending limb and back into the ascending one. The net effect is to retain only solute, and not water, in the interstitium of the medulla. This process coupled with the resorption of solute from the ascending loop of Henle results in an interstitium which is hypertonic, thus, causing water to be absorbed from the descending loop and the collecting tubule.

About 90% of the glomerular filtrate is reabsorbed by the time it reaches the distal tubule (Wilson 1975). The main function of the distal and collecting tubules is the adjustment of the pH, osmolality, and electrolyte content of the urine, as well as the regulation of those substances still present in the filtrate. Potassium, ammonia, and hydrogen ions are secreted by this portion of the nephron, and sodium and bicarbonate are reabsorbed by the same mechanism as in the proximal tubule. Potassium ions are also exchanged for sodium ions, and this exchange is enhanced by aldosterone which is secreted by the adrenal cortex. The ammonia that is secreted combines with hydrogen ions to form ammonium ions ($NH_3^+ + H^+ = NH_4^+$) and this helps to regulate the hydrogen ion (H^+) concentration of the urine. In the collecting duct, urea is also reabsorbed.

The absorption of water in the distal portion of the nephron is regulated by antidiuretic hormone (ADH) which is secreted by the pituitary gland. When the body needs to conserve water, ADH is secreted, and the walls of the distal and collecting tubules are made very permeable, thereby allowing water to be reabsorbed. If the body has excess water, less ADH is produced, the walls of the tubules become less permeable, and the volume of excreted urine increases.

Of the approximate 120 ml/min that was filtered at the glomerulus, only an average of 1 ml/min is finally excreted as urine. This quantity can range from 0.3 ml in dehydration to 15 ml in excessive hydration. For an adult the normal average daily volume of urine is about 1200–1500 ml, with more urine produced during the day than at night. However, the normal range may be from 600–2000 ml/24 h (Bradley et al. 1979). *Polyuria* is an abnormal increase in the volume of urine (>2500 ml), as in diabetes insipidus and diabetes mellitus. *Oliguria* is a decrease in urinary volume, such as occurs in shock and acute nephritis. In an adult it is frequently defined as being <500 ml/24 h (Wagoner and Holley 1978, Muth 1978) or <300 ml/m²/24 h. The term *anuria* designates the complete suppression of urine formation, although in the wider sense of the term it is sometimes defined as being <100 ml/24 h during 2 to 3 consecutive days, in spite of a high fluid intake (Rényi-Vámos and Babics 1972).

The main constituents of urine are water, urea, uric acid, creatinine, sodium, potassium, chloride, calcium, magnesium, phosphates, sulfates, and ammonia. In 24 hours the body excretes approximately 60 g of dissolved material, half of which is urea (Race and White 1979). In some pathologic conditions, certain substances, such as ketone bodies, protein, glucose, porphyrins, and bilirubin, appear in large quantities. Urine can also contain structures such as casts, crystals, blood cells, and epithelial cells.

Some of the renal disorders that a urinalysis can help in diagnosing include: *cystitis,* which is the inflammation of the bladder; *nephritis,* which is the inflammation of the kidney and can either be present with bacterial infection (*pyelonephritis*), or without infection (*glomerulonephritis*); and *nephrosis,* which is the degeneration of the kidney without inflammation.

Collection of Specimen

The performance of an accurate urinalysis begins with the proper collection technique. There are several methods available, depending on the type of specimen needed.

The first important step is the use of a clean, dry container. Disposable containers are preferred by most laboratories, since they avoid the possibility of contamination from improperly washed glass urine bottles. Samples that are to be cultured must be collected in a sterile container. If the specimen is being collected into a bedpan first, then the bedpan must also be sterile.

Methods

One method frequently used is that of collecting the entire voided sample. The problem with this method is that the specimen cannot be used for bacterial examination. Also, in female patients the sample is often contaminated with vaginal discharge.

Catheterization of the bladder is sometimes necessary to obtain a suitable specimen. This method may be used if the patient is having difficulty voiding. It can also be used in a female patient to avoid vaginal contamination, especially during menstruation. However, since this procedure carries with it the possibility of introducing organisms into the bladder which may, in turn, cause infection, it should not be routinely used for the collection of culture specimens.

Suprapubic aspiration of the bladder is sometimes used in place of catheterization for obtaining a single urine sample. It involves the insertion of a needle directly into the distended bladder. This technique avoids vaginal and urethral contamination and can also be useful in getting urine from infants and small children. The specimen obtained by this method can also be used for cytology studies.

The "clean-catch" or clean-voided midstream specimen is usually the method of choice. It is easy to perform and it provides a sample that can be used for bacteriologic examination as well as for routine urinalysis. Prior to collection, the external genitalia are thoroughly cleansed with a mild antiseptic solution. During the collection the initial portion of the urine stream is allowed to escape while the midstream portion is collected into a sterile container.

Women should spread the labia apart while voiding. The final portion of the urine flow is also discarded.

This procedure can be modified if the specimen is not needed for bacterial examination. The midstream collection, without prior cleansing or the use of a sterile container, provides a satisfactory sample for routine urine testing.

In order to obtain suitable specimens from infants and small children, pediatric urine collectors which are attached to the genitalia, are available. These collectors are soft and pliable and cause little discomfort to the patient. As in all urine collections, however, care must be taken to avoid fecal contamination.

One technique that has been used by some nursing personnel for obtaining specimens from infants and which is entirely unsatisfactory, is the practice of squeezing out diapers, especially the disposable diapers. The resulting specimen consists of filtered urine and diaper fibers (see Fig. 3-62); most of the important sediment structures remain in the diaper.

Preservation

Ideally, the specimen for routine urinalysis should be examined while fresh. If this is not possible, then it should be refrigerated until examined. Specimens left at room temperature will soon begin to decompose, mainly due to the presence of bacteria in the sample. Urea-splitting bacteria produce ammonia, which then combines with hydrogen ions to produce ammonium, thereby causing an increase in the pH of the urine. This increase in pH will result in the decomposition of any casts which may be present, because casts tend to dissolve in alkaline urine. If glucose is present, the bacteria may use it as a source of energy which could then result in a false-negative test for glycosuria.

Even if bacterial contamination is not present, some urinary components such as blood cells and casts still tend to deteriorate on standing. However, if the pH of the sample is low and the specific gravity is high (>1.015), deterioration will take longer to occur.

There are times when a urine specimen for an R+M must be saved for a longer period of time than is recommended. This is a common occurrence when specimens are sent to commercial laboratories for analysis. There are several chemical preservatives that can be added to the routine urinalysis specimen but most of them interfere in some way with the testing procedure. For this reason, the routine use of preservatives is not recommended.

Preservatives which can be used for the random R+M specimen include: 1) Toluene (2 ml/100 ml urine). This preservative is good for chemical constituents but it is not effective against bacteria already present in the urine. Because it floats on the surface of the urine, it may be difficult trying to separate the preservative from the specimen for testing; 2) Formalin (1 drop/30 ml urine). This is a good preservative for the urinary sediment but if used in too large a concentration it will precipitate protein (Krupp et al. 1979) and will give a false-positive test for reducing substances; 3) Thymol (1 small crystal). Thymol interferes with the acid precipitation test for protein; 4) Preservative tablets (1 tablet/30 ml urine). These commercially available tablets usually act by releasing formaldehyde. At this concentration the formaldehyde will not interfere with the test for reducing substances, but higher concentrations will result in false positives. Formaldehyde tablets increase the specific gravity by 0.005/1 tablet/30 ml (Bradley et al. 1979); 5) Chloroform. This chemical has been used for inhibiting bacterial growth, but it is not recommended for the R+M specimen because it causes changes in the characteristics of the cellular sediment (Race and White 1979).

Timing

A random sample is usually sufficient for the performance of most urinary screening tests; but, since the first specimen voided in the morning is more concentrated, it is usually the specimen of choice. Samples collected randomly during the day are sometimes so dilute due to increased fluid consumption that they tend to give a false picture of the patient's health.

There are some tests that are best if performed on specimens obtained at certain times of the day. For example, glycosuria is more readily detected on samples taken 2 to 3 hours after eating, while urobilinogen is best evaluated in a specimen collected in the early afternoon.

Since urinary substances are excreted in varying concentrations throughout the day, it is necessary to collect timed specimens in order to accurately quantitate some substances such as creatinine, glucose, total protein, electrolytes, hormones, and urea. The most commonly used sample is the 24-hour specimen. In this procedure, the patient empties the bladder and discards the urine. This is usually done about 8 a.m. All urine is collected for 24 hours thereafter, including the sample at 8 a.m. the next day. The container that is used for the 24-hour specimen should be kept in the refrigerator during the entire collection period. Various chemical preservatives may need to be added to the collection container depending on the substance to be tested. For some tests, such as creatinine and protein, refrigeration alone is sufficient.

In order to get an accurate test result, it is important that all urine excreted during the timed period be collected. It is also important that the timing be exact.

Because of the difficulty that is sometimes encountered when doing 24-hour collections, doctors sometimes order 12-hour or 2-hour timed specimens. However, if not properly collected, these can give misleading results.

Examination of Physical Characteristics

As previously mentioned, the routine urinalysis includes the examination of: 1) physical characteristics, such as color, appearance, and specific gravity; 2) chemical characteristics, including pH, protein, glucose, ketones, occult blood, and sometimes bilirubin, urobilinogen, and nitrite; and 3) microscopic structures in the sediment.

The sample that is sent for an R+M, whether it is a random or a first morning specimen, should be at least 15 ml in volume. When necessary, such as in the case of young children, the procedure can be performed on smaller volumes, but 10–15 ml is preferred. If only one specimen has been sent to the lab for both bacteriology and urinalysis studies, the sample must be cultured first before an R+M is done.

Character

For centuries the visual characteristics of urine have been used by physicians as diagnostic tools. With the progress of medical science, chemical and microscopic tests now allow for a more thorough interpretation of the urine. For example, the microscopic analysis now reveals the exact cause of turbid or cloudy urine. Chemical procedures for glucose and ketones now offer an explanation for the sweet or fruity odor of some urine samples. Chemical tests for blood combined with microscopic examination can usually reveal the cause of red urine.

Since, in most cases, little more information is added by reporting urine color or appearance in addition to all of the other routine procedures, some labs no longer include these in the regular urinalysis report.

COLOR

Normal urine has a wide range of color which is mainly determined by its concentration. This color may vary from a pale yellow to a dark amber, depending on the concentration of the pigments urochrome and, to a lesser extent, urobilin and uroerythrin. The more pigment there is, the deeper the color will be. There are, however, many factors and constituents that can alter the normal urine color. These include medications and diet as well as various chemicals that can be present in disease. Table 1-1 lists some of the substances which may influence the color of urine. This table should not be considered as an all-inclusive list, for there are numerous drugs which are capable of changing the color of urine. It should be noted that the pH of the urine influences the color that many chemicals produce. Also, there may be several coloring factors present in the same urine, which may result in a different color than that expected.

Very pale or colorless urine is very dilute and can result from

Substances That May Color the Urine TABLE 1-1

	Pathologic	Non-Pathologic
White	chyle pus (many WBCs)	phosphates
Yellow to Orange	bilirubin urobilin	acriflavine Azo-Gantrisin carrots concentrated urine food color nitrofurantoin Pyridium quinacrine riboflavin rhubarb senna serotonin sulfasalazine
Pink to Red	hemoglobin myoglobin porphobilin porphyrins red blood cells	aminopyrine antipyrine beets (anthocyanin) bromosulfophthalein cascara diphenylhydantoin food color methyldopa phenacetin phenolphthalein phenolsulfonphthalein phenothiazine Pyridium senna
Red to Brown to Purple	porphobilin porphobilinogen uroporphyrin	
Brown to Black	bilirubin homogentisic acid indican melanin methemoglobin myoglobin phenol p-hydroxyphenyl– pyruvic acid porphyrins	chloroquine hydroquinone iron compounds levodopa methyldopa metronidazole nitrofurantoin quinine resorcinol
Blue to Green	biliverdin *Pseudomonas* infection	acriflavine amitriptyline Azure A creosote Evan's blue methylene blue phenyl salicylate thymol tolonium triamterene vitamin B complex

high fluid consumption, diuretic medication, natural diuretics such as coffee and alcohol, and in such disease states as diabetes mellitus and diabetes insipidus.

The most common cause of red urine is the presence of red blood cells (hematuria). Red urine may also be due to the presence of free hemoglobin (hemoglobinuria), myoglobin (myoglobinuria), or large amounts of uroerythrin which can occur in acute febrile disease. In some types of porphyrinuria, the urine may have a red or a port-wine color, or it may be red only if left standing. In alkaline urine, the dye phenolsulfonphthalein, which is used in tests of kidney function, can cause a red color. Also, some individuals have an inherited metabolic sensitivity which results in the excretion of red urine after eating beets (Berman 1977). This color is due to the presence of complex pigments called anthocyanins (Bauer et al. 1968).

Urine which contains red cells or heme pigments can actually vary in shades from pink through black. The final color is determined by the amount of RBCs or pigment present, the pH of the urine, and the length of contact between the pigment and the urine. For example, an acid urine which contains hemoglobin will darken on standing because of the formation of methemoglobin. This reaction can occur either *in vivo*, as in the bladder, or *in vitro*, while waiting to be tested.

Another cause of dark brown to black urine is alkaptonuria, a rare disorder that is characterized by the excretion of homogentisic acid in the urine. It is due to the congenital lack of the enzyme homogentisic acid oxidase which mediates an important step in the catabolism of tyrosine and phenylalanine. The urine is normal in color when freshly voided but turns dark on standing or when alkalinized (see Chapter 5).

In patients with malignant melanoma, a colorless pigment called melanogen occurs in the urine. On exposure to light, this chromogen is converted to melanin which is black, thus darkening the urine (see Chapter 5).

Patients with obstructive jaundice will excrete bile pigments such as bilirubin, and the urine will be yellow-brown to yellow-green in color. The green pigment is due to biliverdin, the oxidized product of bilirubin, and if the specimen is left standing, the green color will intensify.

There are several medications and dyes which impart a characteristic color to the urine, but these colors are not clinically significant. These include Pyridium and methylene blue, which are used as urinary antiseptics. Pyridium (phenazopyridine), which also acts as an analgesic in the bladder, gives an orange color to the urine and to any foam that may be present. Methylene blue can make the urine blue or blue-green. The presence of Azure A following the Diagnex Blue test for HCl may also turn urine a blue or blue-green color for several days after the test. Multivitamins and riboflavin can give a bright yellow color. Even food dyes such as those used in candies can be excreted in the urine, thus affecting its color.

Although some labs have eliminated the routine reporting of urinary color, one must not overlook the clues given by this physical characteristic. For example, if bilirubin is not included in the routine urinalysis because of the type of dipstick that is used, but the color of the urine strongly suggests its presence, then a test for bilirubin should be performed and the results reported. This may be the first indication to the physician of the patient's problem. Any grossly abnormal color such as black or brown should always be reported. Red urine which has a negative reading for occult blood should also be reported (porphyrins may be present).

APPEARANCE

Normal urine is usually clear but it may become cloudy due to the precipitation of amorphous phosphates in alkaline urine, or amorphous urates in an acid urine. Amorphous phosphates are a white precipitate which will dissolve when acid is added. Amorphous urates frequently have a pink color from urinary pigments, and they will dissolve if the specimen is heated.

Urine can be cloudy from the presence of leukocytes or epithelial cells, and this can be confirmed by microscopic examination of the sediment. Bacteria can also cause cloudiness, especially if the specimen has been sitting at room temperature. Mucous can give the urine a hazy appearance, and red blood cells can result in a smoky or turbid urine. Fat and chyle give urine a milky color.

There are only a few occasions when the odor of urine is important. Ketones can give urine a sweet or fruity smell. A specimen contaminated with bacteria may have a pungent smell from the ammonia that is produced. The excretion of urine that smells like maple syrup is an indication of a congenital metabolic disorder which has been appropriately named "maple syrup urine disease". The urine of an infant with phenylketonuria is said to have a "musty" or "mousy" odor. A urine odor resembling that of "sweaty feet" is found in isovaleric acidemia or in individuals who have excessive amounts of butyric or hexanoic acid (Greenhill and Gruskin 1976). Hypermethioninemia has been associated with a "rancid butter" or "fishy" odor. Since there are several inherited disorders that are associated with a specific odor, Thomas and Howell (1973) have recommended that the prolonged presence of any strong unusual odor in an infant's urine should lead to a complete biochemical workup.

Specific Gravity

The specific gravity is the ratio of the weight of a volume of urine to the weight of the same volume of distilled water at a constant temperature. It is an indicator of the concentration of dissolved material in the urine; however, it is dependent not only upon the number of particles, but also upon the weight of the particles in the solution. The specific gravity is used to measure the concentrating and diluting power of the kidney in its effort to maintain homeostasis in the body. The concentrating ability of the kidney is one of the first functions to be lost as a result of tubular damage.

The normal range for a random specimen is 1.003–1.035, although in cases of excess hydration the reading may be as low as 1.001 (water is 1.000). The value varies greatly depending on the state of hydration and the urinary volume. Usually the specific gravity rises when the fluid intake is low, and falls when fluid intake is high. Since the specific gravity varies throughout the day, a single random reading may not give the physician sufficient information, so a 24-hour collection may be ordered. The range for a 24-hour specimen is 1.015–1.025.

The specific gravity can be useful in differentiating between diabetes insipidus and diabetes mellitus. Both diseases produce a high urinary volume, but in diabetes insipidus the specific gravity is very low because in this disease there is a deficiency of ADH. In diabetes mellitus, there is a deficiency of insulin and thus an excess of glucose, which exceeds the renal threshold and is excreted in the urine. Glucose molecules are very dense and, therefore, the urine will have a very high specific gravity.

Since the specific gravity is affected by the presence of very dense molecules such as protein and glucose, some authors suggest that a correction be made for the glucose and protein concentration. The correction involves subtracting 0.003 from the specific gravity reading (after temperature correction) for each 1 g/dl of protein, and 0.004 for each 1 g/dl of glucose. There is some question whether this correction is necessary, so few laboratories correct for protein and glucose.

Hyposthenuria is a term that is used to describe a urine with a consistently low specific gravity (<1.007). The specific gravity of the glomerular filtrate is believed to be around 1.007 (Wolf 1962, Bradley et al. 1979), so in hyposthenuria there is a concentration problem. The excretion of urine of unusually high specific gravity is called *hypersthenuria,* and this can result from deprivation of water. *Isosthenuria* refers to a fixed specific gravity of 1.010, which indicates poor tubular reabsorption (1.010 was formerly thought to be the specific gravity of the glomerular filtrate).

Some of the causes of increased specific gravity include: dehydration, proteinuria, glycosuria, eclampsia, and lipoid nephrosis. Specific gravity can also be falsely elevated by the presence of such high density compounds as dextrans and the radiographic dyes used in x rays. Depending upon how soon the urine sample is collected after the x-ray procedure, the specific gravity may be greater than 1.050. Since the kidney is limited in how high it can concentrate the urine, a specific gravity reading of >1.035 should be suspected to be caused by abnormal solutes or dyes.

Diseases which can cause decreased specific gravity include: collagen disease, pyelonephritis, hypertension, protein malnutrition, polydipsia, and diabetes insipidus. Diuretic medication as well as the natural diuretics (coffee, alcohol) will also result in specimens having low specific gravities.

URINOMETER

The urinometer is a hydrometer that is calibrated to measure the specific gravity of urine at a specific temperature, usually at 20°C. It is based upon the principle of buoyancy, so the urinometer will float higher in urine than in water, because urine is denser. Thus, the higher the specific gravity of a specimen, the higher the urinometer will float. When using the urinometer it is necessary to make a temperature correction if the urine temperature is not 20°C. For every 3°C below 20°C, subtract 0.001 from the reading, and for every 3°C above 20°C, add 0.001.

It is necessary, therefore, to allow the urine to reach room temperature before measuring the specific gravity. The urinometer should be checked periodically with distilled water to see if it reads 1.000. If not, then a correction factor will have to be used when taking all readings with that instrument. Periodically, a solution of

Urinometer for measuring specific gravity.

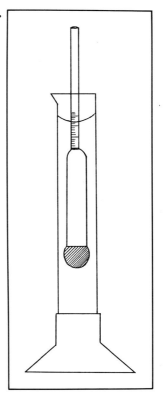

FIGURE 1-3

known specific gravity should also be run, and if the reading is very inaccurate, then the urinometer should be discarded.

The urine is first mixed and then added to a cylinder which usually requires about 15 ml to get a reading (Fig. 1-3). It is necessary to remove any foam which may be present, because the bubbles interfere with the reading of the meniscus. The hydrometer must not come in contact with the bottom or the sides of the cylinder. If it touches the bottom, then add more urine until it floats freely. It is necessary to spin the urinometer so that it will float in the center of the cylinder. Read the bottom of the meniscus while looking at the hydrometer at eye level. The highest reading on most urinometers is 1.035, although some are calibrated to 1.045. If the specific gravity is too high to get a reading, then it is necessary to make a 1:2 dilution of the urine using distilled water. Multiply the last two digits of the reading by 2 to get the true specific gravity. For example, if the dilution reads 1.026, then the specific gravity is 1.052.

REFRACTOMETER

The Total Solids (TS) meter is a refractometer that is specifically designed for measuring the total solids of a solution. The refractometer actually measures the refractive index of the solution, but some models have scales that are calibrated to give readings for specific gravity, total protein, and total solids. Studies have established the relationship between the refractive index and these other measurements (Juel and Steinrauf 1974).

The refractive index is the ratio of the velocity of light in air to the velocity of light in solution. The path of light is deviated when it enters a solution, and the degree of deviation or refraction is proportional to the density of the solution. Like specific gravity, the refractive index also varies with temperature, but the TS meter is temperature-compensated for temperatures between 60°F and 100°F and, therefore, requires no corrections in that range. The TS meter contains a liquid in a sealed chamber in the optical path, and this liquid will also have a refractive index change with temperature, thus compensating for changes in the refractive index of the sample. The chamber also contains an air bubble which allows for the expansion of the liquid, but a bubble trap prevents it from getting into the light path. Figure 1-4 is a schematic diagram of the refractometer and it shows an example of the light path entering and being deviated by the solution and the internal prisms.

The refractometer requires only one drop of specimen, which gives the method an advantage over the urinometer. Because of the large volume of sample that is required for the urinometer, it is often necessary to report out a specific gravity as "qns" (quantity not sufficient), but the refractometer eliminates this problem. To perform the test, first rinse off, then dry the surface of the cover and the prism. Close the cover plate and allow the sample to be drawn under the cover by capillary action. Hold the instrument up to a light source

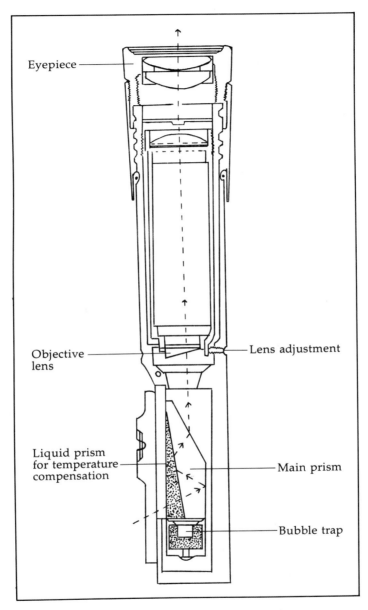

Eyepiece

Objective
lens

Lens adjustment

Liquid prism
for temperature
compensation

Main prism

Bubble trap

Schematic diagram of the Total Solids Refractometer. **FIGURE 1-4**
(Courtesy of the American Optical Company).

and read the specific gravity scale at the light–dark boundary. The scale reads up to 1.035, so specimens that fall off-scale must be diluted.

The zero setting of the instrument should be checked daily with distilled water, but it should rarely, if ever, need adjustment. If the reading is not 1.000, repeat the test before adjusting the setscrew, which moves the objective lens in the light path. This type of instrument does not contain mechanically moving parts and it, therefore, retains its accuracy at any point in the scale. By checking the correctness of a reading at one point against a known standard, accuracy over the entire scale is verified (Goldberg 1965).

SPECIFIC GRAVITY REAGENT STRIPS

The new N-Multistix SG (Ames Co.) contains a reagent area for detecting specific gravity. The test is based on the pKa change of certain pretreated polyelectrolytes in relation to ionic concentration; therefore, the procedure is actually measuring the ionic concentration of the urine, which relates to the specific gravity. The polyelectrolytes in the reagent area contain acid groups which disassociate according to the ionic concentration of the specimen. The more ions in the specimen, the more acid groups will become disassociated, releasing hydrogen ions and causing the pH to change. The reagent area contains a pH indicator (bromthymol blue) which then measures the change in pH. The higher the specific gravity of the urine specimen, the more acidic the reagent area will become.

The colors of the reagent area will range from deep blue-green in urines of low ionic concentration through green and yellow-green in urines of increasing ionic concentration. The color blocks are in increments of 0.005 for specific gravity readings between 1.000 and 1.030.

The chemical nature of the specific gravity reagent strip may cause slightly different results from those obtained with other specific gravity methods when elevated amounts of certain urine constituents are present. Urines that contain glucose or urea in concentrations greater than 1% may have lower specific gravity readings than by other methods, while moderate amounts of protein (100–750 mg/dl) may cause elevated specific gravity readings. Urines that contain radiographic dyes will have lower readings than by other methods, because the iodine in the dye is not ionic and, therefore, it will not react with the reagent. Highly buffered alkaline urines may also cause low readings, so the manufacturer suggests that, for greater accuracy, 0.005 may be added to the readings from urines with pH $\geqslant$6.5 (Ames 1981).

SPECIFIC GRAVITY VS. OSMOLALITY

Urine osmolality and specific gravity are both measures of total solute concentration, but they do not provide the same information. The osmolality depends on the number of particles in the solution, while specific gravity depends on the number and weight of the solutes. Since osmolality is unaffected by the density of such solutes as glucose, protein, dextrans, and radiographic dyes (Race and White 1979), it is a better indicator of the concentrating and diluting abilities of the kidney. But in the past, the osmolality has required more time and more equipment than the specific gravity, which is why it has not been included in the routine urinalysis procedure.

Normally the urinary osmolality and specific gravity have a fairly straight line relationship with approximately 40 mosmoles (milliosmoles) being equal to each unit of specific gravity. Specific gravity values of 1.010, 1.020, and 1.030 are roughly equivalent to 400, 800, and 1200 mosmol/kg water (Sotelo-Avila and Gooch 1976). But in renal disease and in the presence of dense substances, this relationship no longer exists.

The normal adult on a normal diet will produce urine with an osmolality of about 500–850 mosmol/kg water. The normal kidney should be able to produce urine as dilute as 40–80 mosmol/kg water during excessive hydration, and as concentrated as 800–1400 mosmol/kg water during dehydration (Wilson 1975, Bradley et al. 1979). In terminal renal failure the urine osmolality may stay around 285 mosmol/kg, which is the osmolality of plasma and the glomerular filtrate, indicating that the kidney is unable to dilute or concentrate the urine.

The osmolality can be measured either by freezing point or vapor pressure depression. The osmometer which measures the freezing point of a solution is the most frequently used method. A solution which contains 1 osmol or 1000 mosmol/kg water lowers the freezing point 1.86°C below that of water (0°C). So the lower the freezing point, the higher the osmolality. The sample that is needed may range from 0.25 ml to 2 ml depending upon the instrument and the type of cuvette that is used.

2

Chemical Examination

The routine urinalysis includes chemical testing for pH, protein, glucose, ketones, and occult blood. Some laboratories also include tests for bilirubin, urobilinogen, and nitrite, depending on the type of dipstick that is used. It is recommended that a screening test for reducing substances be included in the urinalysis of a child. These procedures are either qualitative (positive or negative) or semiquantitative (e.g. trace through 4+) measurements.

Since the introduction of single and multiple-test reagent strips, test tapes, and tablets, the chemical screening of the urine has become a sensitive and rapid procedure. It is now possible to analyze up to nine different tests in less than 60 seconds. There are two basic brands of dipsticks and each brand has reagent strips which are capable of measuring from one to nine different reactions. In general, this chapter will consider those strips which measure eight determinants, although each company has several strips which can measure the same reaction.

The Ames Company* manufactures the N-Multistix (other reagent strips by Ames also have the suffix "stix"), and the Boehringer Mannheim Corporation† (BMC) makes the Chemstrip 8 (in the USA other strips by BMC are also called Chemstrip). Both dipsticks measure pH, protein, glucose, ketones, occult blood, bilirubin, urobilinogen, and nitrite. Those labs which use Labstix (Ames) and Chemstrip 5 (BMC) do not include bilirubin, urobilinogen, or nitrite. There are some differences between these brands, but they both accurately measure the same constituents (Smith et al. 1977). In this book the term "dipstick" will be used in those instances where the N-Multistix and Chemstrip 8 are the same.

What is a reagent test-strip? Essentially, it is a narrow strip of plastic with small pads attached to it. Each pad contains reagents for a different reaction, thus allowing for the simultaneous determination of several tests. A critical requirement is that the reactions be read at the prescribed time after dipping, and then compared closely with the color chart provided by the manufacturer. In order to get accurate and reliable results with the dipsticks, certain precautions must be taken to help maintain the reactivity of the reagents. The strips must not be exposed to moisture, direct sunlight, heat, or volatile substances, and they should be stored in their original containers. The container should not be kept in the refrigerator nor exposed to temperatures over 30°C. Each vial or bottle contains a dessicant, but the strips should still not be exposed to moisture. Remove only the number of strips needed at a time and then tightly close the con-

* Ames Company, Division of Miles Laboratories, Inc., Elkhart, Indiana.
† Bio-Dynamics/bmc, Division of Boehringer Mannheim, Indianapolis, Indiana and West Germany.

tainer. If the color blocks on the strip do not resemble the "negative" blocks on the color chart, or if the expiration date on the container has past, discard the strips. If the urine specimen has been refrigerated, it should be brought to room temperature before testing.

The procedure for using the dipstick is as follows.

1. Completely dip the test areas of the strip in fresh, well-mixed, uncentrifuged urine and remove immediately. Care should be taken not to touch the test areas.
2. Remove the excess urine from the stick by touching the edge of the strip to the urine container. When using the N-Multistix, hold in a horizontal position after dipping; the Chemstrip 8 should be held vertically.
3. At the correct times, compare the test areas with the corresponding color charts on the container. The strip should be read in good lighting to get an accurate color comparison.

As advances are made in improving the reagent strips, changes may be made in the directions for using them. This may involve a difference in the timing or the reagents that are used, so it is important to always follow the manufacturer's latest directions.

Table 2-1 lists some of the many types of reagent test-strips and tablets that are available for performing single or multiple determinations. As previously mentioned, this chapter will discuss mainly N-Multistix and Chemstrip 8, but some of the other products listed will also be discussed as confirmatory or monitoring procedures.

Even with the widespread use of the rapid and convenient screening procedures, it is still necessary to understand the basic principles of the tests as well as the correct technique to be used. This chapter will include a clinical explanation of the chemical constituents to be tested, the principles behind the tests, an analysis of abnormal results, and several procedures in addition to the dipsticks which can be used as alternative or confirmatory tests. It will also include a brief discussion on quality control and instrumentation in the routine urinalysis laboratory.

Urinary pH

One of the functions of the kidney is to help maintain acid–base balance in the body. To maintain a constant pH (hydrogen ion concentration) in the blood (about 7.40), the kidney must vary the pH of the urine to compensate for diet and products of metabolism. This regulation occurs in the distal portion of the nephron with the secretion of both hydrogen and ammonia ions into the filtrate, and the reab-

Product	pH	Protein	Glucose	Ketones	Blood	Bilirubin	Urobilinogen	Nitrite	Leukocytes	Sp. Gravity
N-Multistix*	x	x	x	x	x	x	x	x		
Chemstrip 8**	x	x	x	x	x	x	x	x		
Multistix*	x	x	x	x	x	x	x			
Chemstrip 7**	x	x	x	x	x	x	x			
Bili-Labstix*	x	x	x	x	x	x				
Chemstrip 6**	x	x	x	x	x	x				
Kova Strip 6***	x	x	x	x	x	x				
Labstix*	x	x	x	x	x					
Chemstrip 5**	x	x	x	x	x					
Hema-Combistix*	x	x	x		x					
Combistix*	x	x	x							
N-Uristix*		x	x					x		
Uristix*		x	x							
Chemstrip GP**		x	x							
Keto-Diastix*			x	x						
Chemstrip GK**			x	x						
Diastix*			x							
Clinistix*			x							
Clinitest*			x							
Chemstrip G**			x							
Tes-Tape****			x							
Albustix*		x								
Hemastix*					x					
Hematest*					x					
Ketostix*				x						
Chemstrip K**				x						
Acetest*				x						
Urobilistix*							x			
Ictotest*						x				
Microstix-Nitrite*								x		
Bac-U-Dip*****								x		
Chemstrip 9**	x	x	x	x	x	x	x	x	x	
Chemstrip L**									x	
N-Multistix SG*	x	x	x	x	x	x	x	x		x

* Ames Co.   ** BMC   *** ICL Scientific
**** Eli Lilly and Co.   ***** Warner-Chilcott Laboratories

sorption of bicarbonate. If sufficient hydrogen ions (H^+) are secreted into the tubule, all of the bicarbonate present will be reabsorbed, but if fewer H^+ are secreted or if an excess of bicarbonate is present, some of the bicarbonate will be excreted in the urine (de Wardener 1967). The continued secretion of H^+ after all bicarbonate has been reabsorbed will drop the pH of the filtrate and result in an acid urine.

The secretion of H^+ in the tubule is regulated by the amount present in the body. If there is an excess of acid in the body (acidosis), more H$^+$ will be excreted and the urine will be acid. When there is an excess of base in the body (alkalosis), less H$^+$ will be excreted and the urine will be alkaline. The hydrogen ions in the urine are excreted as either free H$^+$, in association with a buffer such as phosphate, or bound to ammonia as ammonium ions. The pH of the urine is determined by the concentration of the free H$^+$.

Since pH is the reciprocal of the hydrogen ion concentration, as the H$^+$ concentration increases, the pH decreases or becomes more acidic. As the H$^+$ concentration decreases, the pH increases or becomes more alkaline. The pH of the urine may range from 4.6 to 8.0 but averages around 6.0, so it is usually slightly acidic. There is no abnormal range as such, since the urine can normally vary from acid to alkaline. For this reason, it is important for the physician to correlate the urine pH with other information to determine if there is a problem. In renal tubular acidosis, for example, in spite of a systemic acidosis the urine pH will stay above 6.0 because the tubules are unable to secrete enough hydrogen ions (Douglas and Kerr 1971).

Because normal metabolism produces an excess of acids, the urine is generally acidic. A high protein intake and the ingestion of some fruits such as cranberries will produce an acid urine. Pathologic conditions which will cause acid urine include respiratory acidosis (CO$_2$ retention) and metabolic acidosis as in diabetic ketosis, uremia, severe diarrhea, and starvation. Urinary tract infections caused by *Escherichia coli* will result in an acid urine (Alba 1975). A deficiency of potassium may cause a slightly acid urine even though the person may be in metabolic alkalosis (Bradley et al. 1979).

Because of the excretion of acid into the stomach after eating, the urine normally becomes alkaline or less acidic postprandially, and this is commonly referred to as the "alkaline tide." A diet that is high in vegetables and citrus fruits will also cause an alkaline urine. In respiratory alkalosis (hyperventilation) and in metabolic alkalosis as with vomiting, the urine will have an alkaline pH. Urinary infections caused by such urea-splitting bacteria as *Proteus* and *Pseudomonas* may cause an alkaline urine as high as pH 9.0. This same reaction may occur if a sample that is contaminated with this type of bacteria is left standing before analysis. The bacteria may break down urea into ammonia and the urinary pH will increase. For this reason, a high pH in an old urine has no diagnostic significance.

There are times when it is necessary to regulate the pH of the urine to prevent the formation of kidney stones or to aid in the excretion of a particular substance. Acidifiers such as ammonium chloride, methionine, mandelic acid, and ascorbic acid can be used to suppress chronic bacterial infections (Meyers et al. 1978), or to prevent the formation of alkaline stones including calcium phosphate and calcium carbonate. An alkaline urine can be induced with sodium bicarbonate, potassium citrate, and acetazolamide (a carbonic anhydrase inhibitor). Alkalinization of the urine increases the rate of excretion of salicylate so it is used in the treatment of salicylate poisoning. It is also used to prevent the crystallization and subsequent stone formation of sulfonamides, uric acid, calcium oxalate, and cystine, all of which can precipitate in acid urine. There are also some urinary tract infections that can be treated in this way.

Reagent Test-Strips

Both dipsticks utilize two indicators, methyl red and bromthymol blue, which cover the pH range of 5 to 8.5 or 9. The colors range from orange to yellow and green through blue. The results may be reported in whole units or interpolated to half units (James et al. 1978a). If a more precise reading is needed, measurement may be made using a pH meter with a glass electrode. Some labs report the reaction as "acid", "neutral", or "alkaline", instead of giving numerical values. The pH timing is not critical; the N-Multistix may be read at any time up to 1 minute (Ames 1981), and the Chemstrip should be read within 2 minutes (BMC 1978). However, it is recommended that the pH be read immediately as this will prevent misreadings because of "run-over".

Recent advances have been made to prevent the phenomenon known as "run-over". This term is used to describe what happens when excess urine is left on the stick after dipping, and so the acid buffer from the reagent in the protein area runs onto the pH area. This contamination can cause a false lowering of the pH reading, especially in the case of an alkaline or neutral urine. "Run-over" can sometimes be recognized by the technologist, because the edge nearest the protein area will usually change first. However, if the strip is not observed constantly after dipping, this occurrence can be overlooked. In an effort to minimize this contamination, the new N-Multistix has a hydrophobic inter-pad surface which causes the urine to bead up on it, and thereby reduces "run-over". The design of the Chemstrip is such that a nylon mesh holds the test pads and underlying absorbent papers in place on the plastic strip. The mesh allows for even diffusion of the urine on the test pads, and the underlying paper absorbs excess urine to prevent "run-over".

If pH is the only test needed to be done on a urine specimen, litmus paper or Nitrazine paper* can also be used to obtain an approximate reading.

Protein

The presence of increased amounts of protein in the urine can be an important indicator of renal disease. It may be the first sign of a serious problem and may appear long before other clinical symptoms. There are, however, physiologic conditions such as exercise and fever that can lead to increased protein excretion in the urine in the absence of renal disease. There are also some renal disorders in which proteinuria is absent.

* E.R. Squibb & Sons Division, Olin Mathieson Chemical Corp., New York, N.Y.

In the normal kidney only a small amount of low-molecular-weight (LMW) protein is filtered at the glomerulus. The structure of the glomerular membrane prevents the passage of high-molecular-weight (HMW) proteins including albumin (mol wt = 69,000). After filtration, most of the protein is reabsorbed in the tubules with <150 mg/24 h (or 20 mg/dl) being excreted. In a child the normal excretion is less than 100 mg/m²/24 h (James 1976). The protein that is normally excreted includes a mucoprotein called "Tamm-Horsfall protein" which is not contained in the plasma, but which is secreted by the renal tubules. This protein forms the matrix of most urinary casts (see Chapter 3).

It can then be seen that there are two main mechanisms by which proteinuria can occur: glomerular damage or a defect in the reabsorption process of the tubules. In glomerular damage, the capillary walls become more permeable, thereby allowing large molecules such as albumin to pass through and be excreted in the urine. Some of the conditions which are associated with glomerular proteinuria are glomerulonephritis, systemic lupus erythematosus, hypertension, amyloidosis, pregnancy, diabetes mellitus, and lipoid nephrosis.

In diminished tubular reabsorption the LMW proteins which are normally present in the filtrate are not completely reabsorbed and so they are present in the urine in increased amounts. Such a condition is called tubular proteinuria and can be seen in such diseases as renal tubular acidosis, pyelonephritis, cystinosis, Wilson's disease, Fanconi's syndrome, medullary cystic disease, interstitial nephritis, and rejection of kidney allografts. It should be remembered that it is possible to have glomerular damage and tubular dysfunction together.

Proteinuria may occur as a result of glomerular blood flow changes without necessarily having a structural abnormality. This is seen in congestive heart failure, but the quantity of protein that is lost usually is not more than 500 mg/day (Pryor 1977) to 1 g/day (Douglas and Kerr 1971), unless there is also glomerular damage present.

The concentration of protein in the urine is not necessarily indicative of the severity of renal disease. Proteins with large molecular weights are generally cleared at a lower rate than LMW proteins, and so it may be possible to predict the type of renal disease by the amount and size of the proteins that are present (Wilson 1975).

Severe, mild, and minimal proteinuria all have different significance in evaluating renal disease. Severe proteinuria (>3.5 g/day [Kissner 1979, Papper 1978]) is characteristically seen in patients with glomerulonephritis, lupus nephritis, amyloid disease, lipoid nephrosis, intercapillary glomerulosclerosis, and severe venous congestion of the kidney. In addition to these, moderate proteinuria (0.5–3.5 g/day) is found in many types of renal disease including nephrosclerosis, tubular interstitial diseases, preeclampsia, multiple myeloma, diabetes nephropathy, malignant hypertension, pyelone-phritis with hypertension, and toxic nephropathies such as radiation nephritis. Minimal proteinuria (<0.5 g/day) may be seen with poly-cystic kidneys, chronic pyelonephritis, inactive chronic glomerulo-nephritis, benign orthostatic proteinuria, and some renal tubular diseases.

As previously mentioned, proteinuria may be absent in some cases of renal disease. This absence may sometimes occur during obstruction from kidney stones and tumors, in congenital malformation of the kidney, during certain phases of acute and chronic pyelonephritis (Bradley et al. 1979, Kurtzman and Rogers 1974), and in the nephropathies of hypercalcemia and potassium depletion.

There is a condition which has been called "orthostatic" or "postural" proteinuria. This term is applied to cases where protein is present in the urine when the individual is in an upright position but not when in a recumbent position. These individuals may have unusual anatomical arrangements of the kidney blood vessels, and these vessels probably are compressed when the body is upright (Arnow 1966). Diagnosis of orthostatic proteinuria may be made by collecting the first morning specimen after the patient has been in a horizontal position all night, and then collecting another sample after the person has been standing and walking around for about two hours. Orthostatic proteinuria will be associated with a negative urine protein in the reclining position, and positive protein in the upright position. This is considered a benign condition although there have been a few cases that later showed signs of glomerular damage, and the level of protein excreted rarely exceeds 1 g/day (Bradley et al. 1979). This type of proteinuria may occur in up to 5 percent of healthy adolescents and young adults (Douglas and Kerr 1971).

The presence of protein in the urine does not necessarily mean that a renal problem exists, because it can be found in otherwise healthy individuals. These benign proteinurias can occur with fever, with emotional stress, during salicylate therapy, after exposure to cold, and after strenuous physical exercise. Athletes frequently have protein in their urine and the level increases with the severity of the exercise (Haber et al. 1979). This has been attributed to increased glomerular permeability; however, there may also be a lower level of tubular reabsorption occurring (Bailey et al. 1976). Benign proteinuria has also been reported in cases of non-IgE-mediated food allergies (Crook 1977).

Since protein enters the urine at the level of the kidney, abnormalities and infections of the lower urinary tract usually do not produce proteinuria unless the kidney is also involved or lesions are present. If a urinary tract infection is present in the absence of proteinuria it can be reasonably assumed that the infection is in the lower urinary tract and the kidney is not involved (Lippman 1957, Weller 1971). Of course, urinary infections can occur simultaneously with renal disease, so the presence of proteinuria with pyuria (white blood cells in the urine) does not necessarily mean the infection is in the kidney. Microscopic analysis of the urinary sediment is usually helpful in determining the origin of the infection, especially if casts are present.

Screening Tests

The screening tests for proteinuria are based either on the "protein error of indicators" principle, or on the ability of protein to be precipitated by acid or heat. It is recommended that the dipstick procedure and one of the acid tests be used together (Assa 1977). The reason for this is that the sensitivity differs among these tests. The dipsticks are more sensitive to albumin than other proteins, while the heat and acid tests are sensitive to all proteins. Also, some substances that interfere with the precipitation tests do not interfere with the reaction on the dipstick.

Contamination of the urine with vaginal discharge, semen, heavy mucous, pus, and blood can result in a false-positive reaction with any method that is used (Baker et al. 1966). A very dilute urine can give a false-negative reaction because the concentration of protein fluctuates with the urine flow (de Wardener 1967), therefore, it is important to interpret the protein result by correlating it with the specific gravity. A trace of protein in a dilute urine indicates a greater loss of protein than does a trace amount in a concentrated specimen.

If protein is present in large quantities, the surface tension of the urine will be altered. Agitation of the urine will cause a white foam to develop on the surface of the urine. This occurrence may be helpful as an indicator of proteinuria.

In order to accurately measure the extent of proteinuria and to differentiate the types of protein that are present, confirmed positive screening tests may be followed up by quantitative procedures and/or electrophoretic, immunoelectrophoretic, immunodiffusion, and ultracentrifugation studies.

REAGENT TEST-STRIPS

This colorimetric method is based on the concept known as the "protein error of indicators", a phenomenon which means that the point of color change of some pH indicators is different in the presence of protein from that observed in the absence of protein. Usually the indicator changes from yellow to blue (or green) between pH 3 and pH 4, but in the presence of protein, this color change will occur between pH 2 and pH 3. Therefore, in the presence of protein an "error" occurs in the behavior of the indicator (Free and Free 1974). The indicator used on the N-Multistix is tetrabromphenol blue (3', 3", 5', 5"-tetrabromophenolsulfonphthalein [Bowie et al. 1977]), and the indicator on Chemstrip 8 is 3', 3", 5', 5"-tetrachlorophenol-3, 4, 5, 6,-tetrabromosulfophthalein (BMC 1978).

An acid buffer is added to the reagent area to maintain a constant pH of 3, which in the absence of urine protein produces a yellow color. The development of any green to blue color indicates the presence of protein with the N-Multistix, and any green color indicates protein on the Chemstrip 8. The intensity of the color is proportional to the amount of protein that is present. The timing on the N-Multistix is not critical and it may be read immediately. To get a semiquantitative reading on the Chemstrip 8, take the reading at 60 seconds (or follow the manufacturer's latest directions). The color of the reagent area should be carefully compared with the color chart supplied by the manufacturer. The results are usually reported as negative to 3+ or 4+.

The two brands of dipsticks have different target areas, so they are not clinically interchangeable (Hinberg et al. 1978, James et al. 1978b). The values of the different readings are as follows:

	N-Multistix	Chemstrip 8
Trace	5–20 mg/dl	6–20 mg/dl
1+	30 mg/dl	30 mg/dl
2+	100 mg/dl	100 mg/dl
3+	300 mg/dl	500 mg/dl or more
4+	over 2000 mg/dl	

The values listed for the trace readings are only approximate values. Not all urines with those values will necessarily give a trace reaction. Screening tests should be able to discriminate between normal and abnormal concentrations, but it is possible to get a positive reaction with the dipstick in a normal patient because the trace area is too sensitive (Brody et al. 1971, James et al. 1978b). This situation can occur especially if the specimen is very concentrated.

The dipstick procedure is very sensitive to albumin, the protein that is primarily excreted as the result of glomerular damage or disease (Douglas and Kerr 1971, BMC 1978). Other urine proteins such as gamma globulin, glycoprotein, ribonuclease, lysozyme, hemoglobin, Tamm-Horsfall mucoprotein, and Bence-Jones protein are much less readily detected than albumin (Hinberg et al. 1978, Free and Free 1974, BMC 1978). Therefore, a negative urinary dipstick result does not necessarily rule out the presence of these proteins.

False-positive results: A highly buffered alkaline urine (pH ≥9) which may result from alkaline medication or stale urine, can overcome the acid buffer in the reagent and the area may change color in the absence of protein. If the dipstick is left in the urine for too long, the buffer will be washed out of the reagent, the pH will increase, and the strip will turn blue or green even if protein is not present (Free and Free 1978). Quaternary ammonium compounds which may be used to clean the urine containers will alter the pH and result in a false-positive reaction. With Chemstrip 8, false positives may occur during treatment with phenazopyridine and after the infusion of polyvinylpyrrolidone as a plasma expander (BMC 1978).

False-negative results: These can occur in dilute urines and when proteins other than albumin are present in slightly elevated concentrations.

SULFOSALICYLIC ACID

There are several acids which can be used to precipitate protein and these include sulfosalicylic, trichloroacetic, nitric, and acetic acid. Sulfosalicylic is the most frequently used acid test because it does not necessarily require the use of heat. Different concentrations and proportions of this acid have been used and they each provide different ranges of results. The procedure discussed here uses the solution known as Exton's reagent which is 5% sulfosalicylic acid in a solution of sodium sulfate. Exton (1925) found that adding sodium sulfate to the sulfosalicylic acid causes a more uniform precipitate to be formed.

This procedure is more sensitive than the dipstick, and it is specific for all proteins including albumin, globulins, glycoproteins, and Bence-Jones protein (Bradley et al. 1979). For this reason it is frequently performed along with the dipstick screening test.

EXTON'S REAGENT

Dissolve 88 g of sodium sulfate in 600 ml of distilled water with the aid of heat. Cool. Add 50 g of sulfosalicylic acid and dilute to 1000 ml.

PROCEDURE

1. Centrifuge an aliquot of urine and use the supernatant.
2. Mix equal volumes of supernatant and Exton's reagent.
3. Grade for cloudiness as follows:
   Negative—no cloudiness
   Trace—cloudiness is just perceptible against a black background
   1+—cloudiness is distinct but not granular
   2+—cloudiness is distinct and granular
   3+—cloudiness is heavy with distinct clumping
   4+—cloud is dense with large clumps that may solidify

Many laboratories prefer to get a more accurate reading by comparing the results of the test with a set of graded standards.

False-positive results: These can occur during therapy with tolbutamide, massive doses of penicillin (Andrassy et al. 1978), sulfonamides, and for up to three days following the administration of radiographic dyes (Lippman 1957, Bradley et al. 1979).

False-negative results: A highly buffered alkaline urine can result in a false-negative reaction. A false negative can also occur in a very dilute sample (Wilson 1975).

HEAT AND ACETIC ACID TEST

Proteins are more susceptible to precipitating agents when at the pH of their isoelectric point, which is usually low (Race and White 1979). The method that follows makes use of this principle as well as of the fact that heat renders protein insoluble and causes it to coagulate.

PROCEDURE

1. Centrifuge or filter about 10 ml of urine and decant the supernatant into a pyrex tube. The tube should be about two-thirds full.
2. Hold the bottom of the tube with a test tube holder and boil the upper portion of the tube for about 2 min. (The tube should be held at an angle over the flame, and aimed away from the body.) If cloudiness appears, it may be due to protein, phosphates, or carbonates.
3. Add 3 to 5 drops of 5% or 10% acetic acid, and boil again. The acid will dissolve any phosphates or carbonates which may be causing the cloudiness. It will also lower the pH, bringing it closer to the isoelectric point of proteins; therefore, the cloudiness may increase after addition of the acid due to increased precipitation of proteins.
4. Read the degree of cloudiness of the upper portion of the tube, and report according to the same scale used for the Exton's test.

Some urines remain clear when boiled, but develop cloudiness when the acid is added and the sample is boiled again. This is because metaprotein in alkaline solution is uncoagulable, but when the solution becomes slightly acid or neutral, the protein is precipitated (Baker et al. 1966).

This procedure detects albumin, globulin, and mucoproteins; Bence-Jones protein can be detected if the tube is watched closely during heating. The test is very sensitive and can detect as little as 5 mg/dl of protein, but hemoglobin and myoglobin are not precipitated by this method (Sisson 1976).

False-positive results: Tolbutamide, massive doses of penicillin, and radiographic dyes can result in false-positive reactions (Wilson 1975).

False-negative results: As mentioned previously, hemoglobin and myoglobin are not detected by this method. Highly buffered alkaline urines and very dilute specimens can give false-negative results.

HELLER'S RING TEST

This method may be useful when only a small quantity of urine is available, but the test is not as sensitive as the other precipitation tests. It is also very difficult to attempt to semiquantitate the results (Exton 1925, Race and White 1979).

PROCEDURE. Place a few milliliters of concentrated nitric acid in the bottom of a test tube. Overlay the acid with centrifuged urine by allowing the urine to run slowly down the side of the tube, thus forming two layers of fluid. A *white* precipitate forming at the junction of the liquids within 3 minutes indicates the presence of protein. An attempt may be made to quantitate the density of the ring that is formed.

False-positive results: This test is affected by the same interfering drugs as the heat and acid test. High concentrations of uric acid and urea may give false-positive reactions but these may be overcome by diluting the urine and repeating the test (Baker et al. 1966).

False-negative results: Since this test is not very sensitive, dilute urines may give false-negative results.

The routine use of concentrated nitric acid may be a disadvantage of this test. The procedure for the Robert's ring test is identical to Heller's test, except that the reagent for the former consists of 1 part concentrated nitric acid and 5 parts saturated magnesium sulfate.

Bence-Jones Protein

Bence-Jones protein consists of dimers of either kappa or lambda light chains from immunoglobulins. This protein was first recognized by Henry Bence-Jones in 1847 because of its unusual solubility properties: it precipitates when heated to $40-60°C$ but becomes soluble again when boiled (Stryer 1975). The molecular weight of the protein is small, around 44,000 (Weller 1971), so it is easily filtered through the healthy glomerulus.

In order to understand the process whereby free light chains are excreted in the urine, it is necessary to trace the source of the production of these chains. In certain diseases a malignant clone of immunoglobulin-producing immunocytes is formed (Erslev and Gabuzda 1975). All of the cells in the clone are a result of the proliferation of a single cell, and therefore they have identical properties. These cells will produce a homogeneous immunoglobulin (e.g., all IgG or all IgA) and/or a single type of free light chain, either kappa or lambda. An imbalance in the production rates of the subunits (light and heavy chains) which make up the immunoglobulin molecule can result in the overproduction of light chains which will be filtered at the glomerulus and excreted in the urine (Bence-Jones protein). But this all depends upon the relative quantities of light and heavy chains which the clone produces.

Three types of abnormalities can occur. First, the clone can produce equal amounts of one type of light chain and one type of heavy chain. These will combine to form a homogeneous immunoglobulin which can be detected as a monoclonal spike on the serum electrophoretic pattern. Since no excess light chains are produced, none will be present in the urine (no Bence-Jones protein). Secondly, the clone may produce more light chains than heavy chains. The light chains will combine with all of the available heavy chains and the resulting immunoglobulin can again be detected by serum electrophoresis. The excess light chains will be excreted in the urine (Bence-Jones protein). In the third type, the clone produces only the homogeneous light chains without any heavy chains. Serum electrophoresis will show no monoclonal spike since no homogeneous immunoglobulin molecules can be formed. All of the light chains will be excreted in the urine unless there is renal insufficiency. The urine will therefore contain large quantities of Bence-Jones protein and this can best be identified by a spike on the urine electrophoretic pattern (Boggs and Winkelstein 1975).

Multiple myeloma, a disease in which there is a malignant proliferation of plasma cells, usually in the bone marrow, is the disease most frequently associated with Bence-Jones protein. It is estimated that 50 to 80 percent of patients with multiple myeloma will have Bence-Jones protein in their urine. The remaining cases can be diagnosed by serum electrophoresis or immunoelectrophoresis which can detect the monoclonal immunoglobulin (Eastham 1976).

Bence-Jones proteinuria is not specific for multiple myeloma but can also be found in cases of lymphoma, macroglobulinemia, leukemia, osteogenic sarcoma, amyloidosis, and other malignancies (Balant and Fabre 1978). The daily urinary excretion of light chains may vary from less than 1 g/day to 15 to 20 g/day (Erslev and Gabuzda 1975). With multiple myeloma, however, it is characteristic that if Bence-Jones protein is present, it will appear in large quantities (de Wardener 1967). After prolonged Bence-Jones proteinuria the glomerular membrane may become more permeable to larger proteins, and because of the large demand for protein reabsorption, the tubule cells degenerate (Bradley et al. 1979), so normal serum proteins, albumin, and globulin will also appear in the urine (Lippman 1957).

Testing for Bence-Jones proteinuria is not part of the routine urinalysis but this protein may be accidentally recognized in the heat and acid test. If a request is made for Bence-Jones protein, the sulfosalicylic acid test may be performed first as a screening test for all proteins. If the results are negative, then no Bence-Jones protein is present, but if positive results are obtained, then further testing is required to determine if the precipitation is due to Bence-Jones or other proteins. The best method for detecting the presence of these light chains is by protein electrophoresis and immunoelectrophoresis using specific antisera on a urine specimen that has been well concentrated, usually by dialysis (Pruzanski 1975). There are two other screening procedures that can be used, but they are not as reliable as electrophoresis. One method is based on the protein's unusual solubility properties, while the other is a precipitation test using toluene sulfonic acid (TSA).

HEAT PRECIPITATION TEST

Bence-Jones protein precipitates at temperatures between 40° and 60°C (56°C optimum), but redissolves again at 100°C. Upon cooling, the precipitate will reappear around 60°C and will dissolve again below 40°C.

PROCEDURE
1. Place several milliliters of centrifuged urine in a test tube and acidify to pH 5.0 to 5.5 using 10% acetic acid.
2. Heat for 15 minutes in a 56°C water bath. If a precipitate forms, it is indicative of Bence-Jones protein.
3. If precipitation occurs, place the tube in a boiling water bath and allow to boil for 3 minutes. A decrease in precipitation is due to the presence of Bence-Jones protein, whereas an increase in precipitation is due to other proteins.
4. If an increase in precipitation occurs at 100°C, filter the urine *while it is hot* to remove the interfering proteins. The Bence-Jones protein will be in solution at that temperature and will, therefore, remain in the filtrate.
5. Upon cooling, the Bence-Jones protein will reappear in the filtrate at approximately 60°C and will dissolve again below 40°C.

False-negative results: A very heavy precipitation of Bence-Jones protein at 56°C may not redissolve on boiling, so the procedure should be repeated on diluted urine. If the sample needs to be filtered in step #4, it must remain above 70°C during filtration or else the Bence-Jones protein will begin to precipitate out and will remain in the filter.

TOLUENE SULFONIC ACID TEST

TSA reagent precipitates Bence-Jones protein and can detect as little as 0.03 mg/ml (Race and White 1979). It will not precipitate albumin, but globulins will give a positive test if present at concentrations greater than 500 mg/100 ml (Krupp et al. 1979).

TSA REAGENT
p-Toluene sulfonic acid—12 g
Glacial acetic acid—q.s. to 100 ml

PROCEDURE
1. Place 2 ml of clear urine in a test tube.
2. Add 1 ml TSA reagent by allowing it to flow slowly down the side of the tube. (Take 15 to 30 seconds to add the reagent.)
3. Flick the tube with a finger to mix.
4. A precipitate forming within 5 minutes indicates the presence of free light chains.

Glucose and Other Reducing Substances

The presence of significant amounts of glucose in the urine is called glycosuria (or glucosuria). The quantity of glucose that appears in the urine is dependent upon the blood glucose level, the rate of glomerular filtration, and the degree of tubular reabsorption. Usually glucose will not be present in the urine until the blood level exceeds 160–180 mg/dl, which is the normal renal threshold for glucose (Weller 1971). When the blood glucose exceeds the renal threshold, the tubules cannot reabsorb all of the filtered glucose, and so glycosuria occurs. Normally this level is not exceeded even after the ingestion of a large quantity of carbohydrate. A small amount of glucose may be present in the normal urine, but the fasting level in an adult is only about 2–20 mg of glucose per 100 ml of urine (Krupp et al. 1979).

To understand the presence of glucose in the urine, it is best to first review the source of the glucose that is in the blood. There are three main sources of blood glucose: 1) the digestion of starches and carbohydrates produces glucose which is absorbed from the intestine; 2) gluconeogenesis, which is the conversion of noncarbohydrate precursors into glucose, i.e., protein and fat; and 3) glycogenolysis, the hydrolysis of glycogen which is stored in the liver (Henry 1974).

The main reason for glycosuria is an elevated blood glucose level which is called hyperglycemia. Diabetes mellitus is the most common disease that causes hyperglycemia. This disease results either from a defect in the production of insulin or from the inhibition of the action of insulin. Since insulin is required for the proper utilization of glucose, the result is an upset in not only the metabolism of carbohydrates, but also of fat and proteins. When the hyperglycemia persists, the glucose molecules in the urine have an osmotic diuretic effect which results in the loss of large volumes of water and electrolytes. For this reason, polyuria, polydipsia (an increase in thirst [due to fluid loss]), and polyphagia (an increase in hunger [due to loss of glucose and other nutrients]) are characteristic of diabetes mellitus. The presence of glycosuria is not by itself diagnostic of diabetes mellitus because there are other causes of glycosuria. Such a diagnosis must be based on glucose tolerance tests.

There are various other causes of hyperglycemia which will result in glycosuria. If a large amount of carbohydrate is taken into the digestive tract at one time, sugar will pass from the intestinal tract into the bloodstream faster than the liver can remove it. This type is referred to as alimentary glycosuria, and it can also occur if a high-caloric meal is ingested after fasting for several days, because the body's tolerance to glucose is lowered. Hyperglycemia of this type is transitory.

Stress and anxiety may result in an increased output of

epinephrine and glucocorticoid cortisol. Epinephrine mobilizes glucose from its glycogen stores in the liver, and cortisol stimulates gluconeogenesis and also decreases the ability of the body to use glucose (D'Eramo and McAnear 1974). Cushing's syndrome also displays an excessive production of glucocorticoids.

Pancreatic diseases which result in a decrease in the production of insulin will also cause elevated glucose levels. Some of the other miscellaneous causes of hyperglycemia may include hyperthyroidism, infection, asphyxia, gastrectomy, myocardial infarction, general anesthesia, brain tumors, cerebral hemorrhage, obesity, and glycogen storage diseases. The administration of thiazide diuretics or steroids can also result in the impairment of carbohydrate metabolism with resulting hyperglycemia (Waife 1979).

Glycosuria is never due to an increased glomerular filtration rate (de Wardener 1967), but if the filtration rate is very low, all of the filtered glucose will be reabsorbed even though the plasma concentration may be elevated (Pitts 1968). This can explain the reason why a patient who is in a diabetic coma may occasionally not have any measurable glycosuria. The filtration rate may be greatly reduced because of extreme dehydration. A patient who has had diabetes for many years may develop a high renal threshold for glucose. This is probably due to a decreased glomerular filtration rate which can occur with diabetic nephropathy (Waife 1979, Pitts 1968).

The third factor which can affect glycosuria is a defect in the reabsorptive ability of the renal tubules and it results in what is termed renal glycosuria. Some individuals have a congenitally low renal threshold level. This condition is benign, but studies must first confirm the presence of normal blood glucose levels along with the glycosuria. For some reason these individuals are not capable of reabsorbing as much glucose as is the average person. Renal glycosuria may coexist with diabetes in children, and the child may be constantly glycosuric despite hypoglycemic blood levels (Waife 1979). In these cases, treatment must be based on blood glucose levels. The glycosuria which may be present in pregnancy is also believed to be due to a lowered renal threshold for glucose reabsorption (de Wardener 1967).

Besides the benign type of glycosuria, there are other tubular defects that result in the decreased ability to reabsorb glucose. These can include Fanconi's syndrome, cystinosis, and heavy-metal poisoning.

Glucose is not the only sugar that may appear in the urine. Others which may be present include galactose, lactose, fructose, maltose, mannose, and pentoses. Of these, galactose which occurs in infants with a congenital metabolic defect, is the most significant. Lactose may occur in the urine of nursing women and during late pregnancy. It may also be found in the urine of premature infants (Stedman 1976). All of these sugars, including glucose, are reducing substances and so those procedures which are based on the ability of glucose to reduce copper will also detect these sugars if they are present. Any other reducing substances which can occasionally be found in the urine such as dextrins, homogentisic acid, and glucuronates will also give positive reduction tests.

There are two basic types of tests which are used to screen or monitor glycosuria. The procedures which use the enzyme glucose oxidase are specific for glucose, while the copper reduction tests will detect any reducing substance. As with all screening procedures, a positive test result should be correlated with other findings. The interpretation of a positive glucose test should be based on the other screening tests, including specific gravity, ketones, and albumin. But more importantly, a correlation must be made with the blood glucose level, as well as the case history, family history, and clinical picture. A previously undiagnosed glycosuria should be followed up by such studies as a glucose tolerance test, 2-hour postprandial glucose, and fasting blood sugar. A positive reducing substance other than glucose can best be differentiated by either thin-layer or paper chromatography.

Glucose Oxidase Test

Paper strips and dipsticks that are impregnated with the enzyme glucose oxidase detect only glucose. These strips use the following double sequential enzyme reactions:

$$\text{glucose} + O_2 \xrightarrow{\text{glucose oxidase}} \text{gluconic acid} + H_2O_2$$

$$H_2O_2 + \text{chromogen} \xrightarrow{\text{peroxidase}} \text{oxidized chromogen} + H_2O$$

The chromogen that is used varies among the different reagent strips. Table 2-2 lists the main reagent strips that are used, along with the corresponding chromogen, the color change that will occur, and the values of the different color blocks which are marked on the dipstick or paper strip container (these are subject to change by the

TABLE 2-2		Reagent Strips for Screening or Monitoring Urinary Glucose					
Product	Chromogen	Color Change	% Concentration				
			Trace	1+	2+	3+	4+
N-Multistix*	Potassium iodide	blue-green-brown	$1/10$	$1/4$	$1/2$	1	2
Chemstrip 8**	Cl-APAC	yellow-brown	—	$1/10$	$1/4$	1	—
Tes-Tape***	O-Tolidine	yellow-green-blue	—	$1/10$	$1/4$	$1/2$	2
Clinistix*	O-Tolidine + red dye	pink-purple	—	S	M	H	—
Diastix*	Potassium iodide	blue-green-brown	$1/10$	$1/4$	$1/2$	1	2
Chemstrip G**	Cl-APAC	yellow-brown	—	$1/10$	$1/4$	1	2

* Ames Co.
** BMC
*** Eli Lilly and Co.

S = Small
M = Moderate
H = Heavy

manufacturer). The N-Multistix and the Chemstrip 8 are used as screening tests in the routine urinalysis. The other methods that are listed can be used by diabetics to monitor their urine glucose levels. The timing to be used for each product that is listed will vary according to the product. It is imperative that the exact timing as well as all other directions be followed carefully. For example, Chemstrip 8 requires reading of the glucose test at 60 seconds for semiquantitative values, but since the color reaction is kinetic and if elevated will continue to react after 60 seconds, a reading taken after that time will be falsely elevated. On the other hand, the Chemstrip G (BMC) uses the same kinetic color reaction as the Chemstrip 8, but the reaction must be allowed to reach completion before the color comparison is made. (The color chart is different from that of the Chemstrip 8.) So values that are less than 100 mg/dl (0.1%) may be read at 1 minute, but higher values should be read at 5 minutes (BMC 1978).

False-positive results: No known constituent of urine will give a false-positive enzyme test, but if the urine specimen is contaminated with peroxide or hypochlorite, a false-positive reaction may occur.

False-negative results: High urinary concentrations of ascorbic acid (vitamin C) can inhibit the enzymatic reaction which will result in a reduced or false-negative reading. The ascorbic acid will be oxidized by the hydrogen peroxide in the second part of the enzyme reaction, and will, therefore, compete with the oxidation of the chromogen, resulting in the inhibition of the color formation (Brandt et al. 1977). The ingestion of a normal amount of vitamin C usually presents no problem, but the recent interest in the self-prescription of large doses of vitamin C (2–15 g/day) to prevent or cure the common cold has created a potential problem. Large concentrations of urinary ascorbic acid can also occur with the parenteral administration of vitamin C or antibiotics that contain ascorbic acid as a stabilizing agent (e.g., tetracycline). If vitamin C interference is suspected, a repeat test should be performed at least 24 hours after the last intake of ascorbic acid.

With the N-Multistix, a specific gravity greater than 1.020, particularly in combination with a high pH, may reduce the sensitivity of the glucose test, which can result in false negatives at low concentrations of glucose. Moderately high ketone levels (40 mg/dl) can also reduce the sensitivity and may cause false negatives with glucose levels of 100 mg/dl (Court et al. 1972). It would be unusual, however, to have such a high level of ketones in a diabetic with only a small amount of glucose (Ames 1979).

With the Chemstrip 8, changes in pH within the range of pH 4–8 do not affect the color reaction. Urinary concentrations of ketones as high as 250 mg/dl have been shown not to interfere with the Chemstrip semiquantitative glucose test (BMC 1978).

The glucose oxidase methods are more sensitive to solutions of aqueous glucose than to glucose in urine, therefore, they are more sensitive to dilute urine than concentrated urine (Free and Free 1974). Also, because these methods are enzymatic, urines which have been refrigerated must be first brought to room temperature before accurate testing can be done.

Screening for Reducing Substances

The copper reduction tests, Clinitest and Benedict's, are used to test for glucose but they will also detect any other reducing substance which may be present. These procedures can be used to screen for reducing substances, to monitor diabetic urines, or as a confirmatory test for a positive glucose oxidase test. A test for reducing substances should be included in the routine urinalysis of all pediatric patients. This will provide for the early detection of those metabolic defects which are characterized by the excretion of sugars, e.g., galactosemia.

To determine if a positive copper reduction test is due to the presence of glucose or another reducing substance, both the glucose oxidase test and the reduction test must be performed and a correlation made of the results. Following is a list of the possible results along with the interpretation.

Glucose Oxidase	Copper Reduction	Interpretation
+	+	glucose
−	+	nonglucose reducing substance (unless ascorbic acid is present)
+	−	small quantity of glucose

The third possibility of a positive enzyme test but a negative reducing test, can occur when only a small amount of glucose is present, because the enzyme test can measure as little as 0.1% but the Clinitest reducing test can only detect 0.25%.

The methods used to detect reducing substances are based on the fact that in strongly alkaline solutions and in the presence of heat, reducing sugars will reduce cupric ions to cuprous oxide. The reaction produces a color change of blue through green to orange (or red), depending upon the amount of reducing substances present in the urine.

CLINITEST TABLETS

Clinitest (Ames Co.) is a self-heating method for the semiquantitative determination of reducing substances in the urine. The tablet contains the following reagents: copper sulfate, citric acid, sodium hydroxide, and sodium carbonate. When placed in a mixture of water and urine, the tablet is rapidly dissolved by the action of sodium carbonate and citric acid which act as effervescents. The sodium hydroxide provides the alkaline medium necessary for the reaction, and the heat required is provided by the reaction of sodium hydroxide with water and citric acid. The reducing substances in the urine then react with the copper sulfate to reduce the cupric ions to cuprous oxide.

PROCEDURE
1. Place 5 drops of urine into a test tube (or use 0.3 ml).
2. Add 10 drops of water (or 0.6 ml) and mix by shaking.
3. Drop 1 Clinitest tablet into the tube, and observe the complete reaction. Do not shake the tube during the reaction or for 15 seconds after the boiling has stopped. *Warning:* The bottom of the tube will become very hot!
4. At the end of the 15-second waiting period, shake the tube gently and then compare with the color chart that is provided. The test is reported as negative, ¼% (or trace), ½% (1+), ¾% (2+), 1% (3+), or 2% (4+). During the reaction, if the color should rapidly "pass-through" bright orange to a dark brown or greenish-brown, report the result as being greater than 2%.

Clinitest is a very accurate procedure if the manufacturer's directions are carefully followed. Failure to observe the reaction as it takes place will result in a falsely low reading. The "pass-through" phenomenon can occur so rapidly that it can be missed if not observed closely. If measurement beyond 2% is medically desirable, an alternate "2-drop method" is available. This method involves adding only 2 drops of urine to 10 drops of water, but a special color chart must be used. The 2-drop method will allow for quantitation up to 5% but the "pass-through" phenomenon may still occur when very large concentrations of sugar are present.

False-positive results: Nalidixic acid, cephalosporins, probenecid, and the urinary preservatives formalin and formaldehyde if present in large quantities may cause false-positive results. High concentrations of ascorbic acid have been considered to give false-positive results, but recent *in vivo* studies by Smith and Young (1977) and Nahata and McLeod (1978) question whether this is really a problem. The sensitivity of Clinitest (¼%) is such that a number of substances which react positively with Benedict's solution (sensitivity is around 0.05%) will, in most cases, not be present in sufficient quantities to react with Clinitest, e.g., salicylates and penicillin (Ames 1978a).

False-negative results: If all directions for the procedure are followed closely, no false-negative results will occur.

Clinitest is an accurate and reliable test for reducing substances. It has been recommended by Court et al. (1972) as the test of choice for diabetic patients who are ill, when there is poor diabetic control, if ketonuria is present, and during the stabilization of a diabetic.

BENEDICT'S QUALITATIVE TEST

Benedict's test has long been the standard method for detecting glycosuria although it is not specific for glucose. The reaction is very similar to that of Clinitest, with a blue alkaline copper sulfate reagent being reduced to red cuprous oxide precipitate.

REAGENT
Copper sulfate—17.3 g
Sodium or potassium citrate—173 g
Sodium carbonate crystals—200 g
or, anhydrous sodium carbonate—100 g
Distilled water to make 1000 ml

Dissolve the citrate and carbonate in about 700 ml of water with the aid of heat. Filter. Dissolve the copper sulfate in approximately 100 ml of hot water and pour into the citrate–carbonate solution with stirring. Allow to cool before diluting up to 1000 ml with water.

PROCEDURE
1. Place 5 ml of reagent in a test tube.
2. Add 8 drops of urine and mix well.
3. Place in a boiling water bath for 5 minutes or boil over a flame for 1-2 minutes.
4. Allow to cool slowly.

The test is usually graded in intensity according to the following:

Negative—clear blue color, blue precipitate may form
Trace—bluish-green color
1+—green color, green or yellow precipitate
2+—yellow to green color, yellow precipitate
3+—yellow-orange color, yellow-orange precipitate
4+—reddish-yellow color, brick red or red precipitate

This procedure is very sensitive and may be capable of detecting as little as 0.02% (Krupp et al. 1979, Frankel 1963a) or 0.05% (Sisson 1976, Bradley et al. 1979) of reducing substances, and as high as 4% (Race and White 1979). Because of this extreme sensitivity, healthy individuals may show a "trace" reaction.

False-positive results: Benedict's reagent is also reduced by glucuronides and homogentisic acid. Massive doses of various drugs including penicillin, streptomycin, salicylates, oxytetracycline, polyvinylpyrrolidone, dextran, and p-aminosalicyclic acid may also cause a false-positive Benedict's test. The urinary preservatives formalin and formaldehyde are reducing substances and so their presence may result in a false positive. Bradley et al. (1979) state that prolonged boiling during the procedure may also give false-positive results. Heavy proteinuria and heavy urate deposits can also interfere with the test, giving false positives (Lippman 1957). The protein may be removed by precipitating out the protein and then filtering the urine before performing the procedure. For a more complete listing of interfering substances refer to Wirth and Thompson (1965) or Wilson (1975).

False-negative results: Failure to follow the procedure correctly is the only cause of false negatives.

Ketones

Ketone bodies are formed during the catabolism of fatty acids. One of the intermediate products of fatty acid breakdown is acetyl CoA. Acetyl CoA enters the citric acid cycle (Krebs cycle) in the body if fat and carbohydrate degradation are appropriately balanced. The first step in the Krebs cycle is the reaction of acetyl CoA with oxaloacetate to yield citrate. When carbohydrate is not available or is not being properly utilized, all available oxaloacetate will be used to form glucose, and so there will be none available for condensation with acetyl CoA (Stryer 1975). Since acetyl CoA cannot enter the Krebs cycle, it will be diverted to the formation of ketone bodies.

The ketone bodies are acetoacetic acid (diacetic acid), β-hydroxybutyric acid, and acetone. Acetoacetic acid is the first ketone that is formed from acetyl CoA, and the other ketones are formed from acetoacetic acid as follows:

The β-hydroxybutyric acid is formed by reversible reduction, and acetone is formed by a slow spontaneous decarboxylation.

Acetoacetic acid and β-hydroxybutyric acid are normal fuels of respiration and are important sources of energy. In fact, the heart muscle and the renal cortex prefer to use acetoacetate instead of glucose. But glucose is the major fuel of the brain in well-nourished individuals, even though the brain can adapt to utilize acetoacetate in the absence of glucose (Stryer 1975).

Most of the acetone in the body is eliminated via the lungs.

The odor of acetone may be detected in the breath of an individual who has a high level of ketones in the blood.

There are normally small amounts of ketone bodies present in the blood (Weisberg [1974] lists the normal range as 2–4 mg/dl, while Henry [1964] gives 0.5–3.0 mg/dl) and the relative proportion of each is approximately 20% acetoacetic acid, 2% acetone, and 78% β-hydroxybutyric acid. There may, however, be considerable proportional variation among individuals (Mayes 1973). Disorders which are characterized by an altered carbohydrate metabolism can result in an excessive breakdown of fat for use as energy. This, in turn, will cause an increase in the amount of ketone bodies in the blood (ketonemia) and increased levels of ketones in the urine (ketonuria). Ketosis refers to the increase of ketones both in the blood and in the urine. When the capacity of the tissues for utilizing the ketone bodies is exceeded, the excess is excreted in the urine. When the capacity of the kidneys for excreting ketones is exceeded, they accumulate in the blood (Latner 1975, Henry 1974). Ketonuria, therefore, will occur before there is a significant increase of ketones in the blood.

Ketosis can be found in conditions associated with a decreased intake of carbohydrates (starvation), decreased utilization of carbohydrates (diabetes mellitus), digestive disturbances, dietary imbalance (high fat diet, low carbohydrate diet), eclampsia, prolonged vomiting, and diarrhea. Glycogen storage disease (von Gierke's disease) can also result in the excessive production of ketones. Ketosis can occur in thyrotoxicosis, severe prolonged exercise, and fever because there is an increase in metabolism with a resulting requirement for carbohydrate (Latner 1975). An increase in ketones can also occur following ether or chloroform anesthesia (Levinson and MacFate 1969). When the liver is severely damaged by disease or by poisons, carbohydrate cannot be stored in adequate amounts and so fat is burned at an increased rate and ketosis results.

The ketone bodies are mildly toxic, tending to interfere with the excretion of uric acid and to produce a mild depression of the central nervous system (Weisberg 1974). They are able to ionize and to release hydrogen ions and so if they are present in large quantities, acidosis will occur. Acetoacetic acid and β-hydroxybutyric acid combine with sodium bicarbonate, forming sodium salts, carbon dioxide, and water. These sodium salts are then excreted in the urine. Since this causes a decrease in the blood level of sodium bicarbonate, it is another reason for the production of acidosis. Ketoacidosis refers to the acidosis resulting from the presence of ketone bodies.

One of the most important disorders in which ketoacidosis can occur is diabetes mellitus. If the acidosis is severe and if it lasts for a sufficient length of time, the patient becomes drowsy and dull, then lapses into a coma (diabetic coma), and can die if not treated promptly (Arnow 1966). If ketosis occurs in a diabetic, it is a serious sign that the disease is out of control, and the physician must readjust the medication. Such a situation can occur quite readily in juvenile diabetics. Some of the underlying causes of diabetic ketoacidosis include infection, trauma, or failure to take insulin (Howanitz and Howanitz 1979). The presence of large concentrations of glycosuria and ketonuria usually implies that diabetic ketoacidosis is either present or is imminent. Blood glucose levels, ketone levels, and electrolytes should be monitored to determine the course of treatment.

The screening procedures that are used to detect ketonuria do not react with all ketone bodies. Since all three of the ketones are present in the urine and all are equally significant, it is sufficient to detect an increase in any one or two of the ketone bodies. Most procedures will measure diacetic acid (acetoacetic acid) and/or acetone.

There is some question regarding the normal range of ketones in the urine (Henry 1964), but Sisson (1976) lists the range for diacetic acid as up to 2 mg/dl. Hoffman (1970) and Race and White (1979) state that the normal individual on a normal diet can excrete up to about 20 mg of ketone bodies per day. In severe diabetic acidosis, the daily excretion of ketones can reach 40 g/day (Hoffman 1970).

Since acetone is lost into the air if a sample is left standing at room temperature, urines should be tested immediately or refrigerated in a closed container.

Reagent Test-Strips

N-Multistix contains the reagents sodium nitroprusside and an alkaline buffer, which react with diacetic acid in urine to form a maroon color. This dipstick does not react with acetone or β-hydroxybutyric acid (Ames 1981). N-Multistix is read at 15 seconds, and will detect as little as 5–10 mg/dl of diacetic acid. The color change is from buff-pink to maroon and the reaction is reported as either: negative, trace, moderate, or large, or as: negative, 5, 15, 40, 80, or 160 mg/dl (Ames 1981).

With the N-Multistix, false-positive results (trace or less) may occur when the urine specimen is highly pigmented or when it contains large amounts of levodopa metabolites. Some specimens which have both a high specific gravity and a low pH may give false-positive reactions of up to and including "trace" (5 mg/dl) (Ames 1981).

Because of the specificity of the new N-Multistix for diacetic acid, the ketone reagent will not give a positive result with controls which contain acetone.

Chemstrip 8 contains the following reagents: sodium nitroferricyanide, glycine, and an alkaline buffer. The sodium nitroferricyanide and glycine react with diacetic acid and acetone in an alkaline medium to form a violet dye complex. This test-strip is more sensitive to diacetic acid than to acetone, and the reaction does not detect β-hydroxybutyric acid. Chemstrip 8 is read at 60 seconds, and will detect 5–10 mg/dl of diacetic acid and 40–70 mg/dl of acetone. The color change is from beige to violet and the reaction is graded as: negative, 1+ (5–40 mg/dl), 2+ (40–100 mg/dl), or 3+ (>100 mg/dl) (BMC 1978).

Phenylketones may cause a red-orange coloration. Phthalein compounds used in liver and kidney function tests produce a reddish coloration due to the alkalinity of the test zone. These colors, however, are easily distinguishable from the colors obtained with ketone bodies (Bio-Dynamics/bmc 1979a).

Acetest Tablets

The Acetest tablet (Ames Co.) contains sodium nitroprusside, glycine, a strong alkaline buffer (disodium phosphate), and lactose. It can be used to test urine, serum, plasma, or whole blood. Diacetic acid and acetone react with sodium nitroprusside and glycine in an alkaline medium to form a purple color. The lactose in the tablet helps to enhance the color (Tietz 1976). Acetest is about 10 times more sensitive to diacetic acid than to acetone and will not react with β-hydroxybutyric acid. In urine it will detect as little as 5–10 mg/dl of diacetic acid. Bradley et al. (1979) set the detection of acetone at 20–25 mg/dl.

PROCEDURE
1. Place the tablet on a piece of clean, dry white paper.
2. Put 1 drop of urine, serum, plasma, or whole blood directly on top of the tablet.
3. For urine, compare the color of the tablet with the color chart at 30 seconds. For serum or plasma, compare the color after 2 minutes. For whole blood, remove the clotted blood from the tablet after 10 minutes and compare the color of the tablet with the chart.

Results are reported as "small, moderate, or large". In urine, the small color block corresponds to approximately 5–10 mg/dl of diacetic acid, the moderate block is 30–40 mg/dl, and the large block is about 80–100 mg/dl. With serum, plasma, and whole blood, the lowest limit of detection is 10 mg of diacetic acid per 100 ml (Ames 1975a).

Those substances which interfere with the dipsticks will also interfere with the Acetest tablet because the same reaction is involved.

Rothera's Test

Rothera's test is a nitroprusside ring test which is very sensitive to diacetic acid but less sensitive to acetone; β-hydroxybutyric acid is not detected. This method can detect about 1–5 mg/dl of diacetic acid and 10–25 mg/dl of acetone (Bradley et al. 1979).

REAGENTS
1. Rothera's reagent—Pulverize and mix 7.5 g sodium nitro-prusside and 200 g ammonium sulfate.
2. Concentrated ammonium hydroxide.

PROCEDURE   (Bradley et al. 1979)
1. Add about 1 g of Rothera's reagent to 5 ml of urine in a test tube and mix well.
2. Overlay with 1 ml of concentrated ammonium hydroxide.
3. If positive, a red to purple ring will develop within 1½ minutes at the point of contact. Report as follows:
   Negative—no ring or a brown ring
   Trace—faint pinkish purple ring
   2 +—narrow dark purple ring
   4 +—wide dark purple ring

This procedure has, for the most part, been replaced by the reagent dipsticks and Acetest.

Gerhardt's Test

Gerhardt's test is based on the reaction of ferric chloride with diacetic acid to form a port wine or Bordeaux red color. This procedure will not detect either acetone or β-hydroxybutyric acid. It is not a very sensitive test because it can only detect about 25–50 mg/dl of diacetic acid (Henry 1964).

REAGENT
10% ferric chloride—10 g of ferric chloride; q.s. to 100 ml with distilled water

PROCEDURE
1. Place from 3 to 5 ml of urine into a test tube.
2. Add 10% ferric chloride solution drop by drop until all phosphates are precipitated and then add a slight excess of ferric chloride. If diacetic acid is present, a Bordeaux red color will develop.
3. Colors are produced by substances other than diacetic acid, such as blue to red-violet by salicylates, green by phenylpyruvic acid, dark red by aminopyrine, and gray by melanin (Lippman 1957). Phenothiazine drugs also give false-positive reactions. To confirm the presence of diacetic acid, boil another portion of urine for 15 minutes; this will decompose diacetic acid to acetone, which is not detected by ferric chloride. Repeat the test on the boiled sample and if the test is still positive, then diacetic acid is not present but the color is from an interfering substance. If the repeated test is negative, then the color in the original test was due to diacetic acid.

Gerhardt's test is a qualitative procedure and is reported as either positive or negative. Because of the sensitivity of this method, a positive result implies a significant level of ketonuria.

Hart's Test

Hart's test is an indirect method for the detection of β-hydroxybutyric acid in the urine. The first part of the procedure uses boiling to break down the diacetic acid that is present into acetone, and then the acetone is removed by evaporation. Next, the β-hydroxybutyric acid is oxidized to diacetic acid and acetone by the use of peroxide. (Ferric ions or dichromate could also be used.) The diacetic acid and acetone can then be detected by any of the nitroprusside procedures.

PROCEDURE
1. Place 20 ml of urine in a beaker.
2. Add 20 ml of distilled water and a few drops of acetic acid.
3. Boil until the volume is reduced to 10 ml. These steps will remove the diacetic acid and acetone.
4. Dilute to 20 ml with distilled water, mix and divide the contents into 2 equal portions.
5. To one of the portions add 1 ml of hydrogen peroxide, warm gently, and then let cool. This will change the β-hydroxybutyric acid into diacetic acid and some of this will become acetone.
6. Test both portions for diacetic acid and acetone by using any nitroprusside method.
7. If β-hydroxybutyric acid is present, the tube containing the hydrogen peroxide will show a positive reaction. The other tube will show no reaction.

This procedure can be performed on less than 20 ml of urine. If, for instance, 15 ml is used, then add 15 ml of distilled water, evaporate to $7\frac{1}{2}$ ml, and dilute back up to 15 ml.

Occult Blood

The term "occult" means "hidden", and since the methods used to test for blood in the urine are capable of detecting even minute amounts, the test is said to be for occult blood. Another reason for this title is that these procedures actually detect the free hemoglobin from lysed red blood cells. Recent improvements in the dipsticks now allow for the detection of intact red blood cells (RBCs) by causing them to lyse while on the test pad. Formerly, intact RBCs could not be detected. In cases where all of the red cells stayed intact, it was possible to get a negative test for blood even though the microscopic examination revealed the presence of RBCs.

The chemical methods which are used in the routine urinalysis for detecting blood (hematuria) will also detect free hemoglobin (hemoglobinuria) and myoglobin (myoglobinuria). Since the urine is normally free of all of these substances, a positive test for occult blood should be followed by determination of the exact cause and origin of this abnormal finding. A correlation must also be made with the microscopic examination, and this may be done by asking the following questions. Are there red cells present? Does the number of red cells agree with the intensity of the chemical test? Are there red cell casts or hemoglobin casts? Are there empty red cell membranes (ghost cells)? Are there numerous squamous epithelial cells present (possible menstrual contamination)? It should be noted that hematuria, hemoglobinuria, and myoglobinuria can occur either individually or together.

Hematuria

Hematuria is the presence of blood or intact red blood cells in the urine. A urine that is highly alkaline or has a very low specific gravity (<1.007) can cause the red cells to lyse, thus releasing their hemoglobin into the urine. The presence of this type of hemoglobin is still considered to be hematuria as far as the origin is concerned, but it is very difficult to distinguish from true hemoglobinuria. When lysing occurs, the microscopic examination may show the empty red cell membranes which are often referred to as "ghost" cells.

In microhematuria there is such a small amount of blood in the urine that the color of the specimen is unaffected and the hematuria can only be detected chemically or microscopically. On the other hand, gross hematuria alters the color of the urine and is easily visible macroscopically. There is some controversy concerning the number of RBCs that can be present normally, and the number that constitutes microhematuria (Freni et al. 1977). Generally, red blood cells are not found in the normal centrifuged urine, but the finding of 1–2 RBCs per high power field should not be considered abnormal (Wilson 1975, ROCOM 1975, Bradley et al. 1979, Hoffman 1970).

Red cells may enter the urine anywhere from the glomerulus to the urethra. Thus, hematuria can occur in renal (kidney) diseases such as acute glomerulonephritis, which is often referred to as hemorrhagic nephritis because of the frequency with which it is accompanied by hematuria. Some of the other renal diseases that can cause hematuria are: malignant hypertension, polycystic kidney disease, lupus nephritis, infarction, malignant nephrosclerosis, acute infection, renal tumors, renal vein thrombosis, chronic glomerulonephritis, tuberculosis of the kidney, periureteritis, nephrotic syndrome, acute papillary necrosis, hydronephrosis, and damage to the glomerulus such as can occur because of toxins. Renal calculi may cause an intermittent hematuria (Lytton 1977). Trauma to the kidneys frequently results in hematuria which can range from mild to severe; however, the degree of hematuria does not necessarily correlate with the severity of the injury (Bright et al. 1978). The finding of red cells casts in the microscopic examination and/or proteinuria helps to pinpoint the hematuria as originating in the kidney.

Bleeding can also occur in the lower urinary tract. Lytton (1977) states that the most common cause of hematuria is acute cystitis. Other causes include calculi and tumors in the ureter or in the bladder, also trauma, lesions, infections, strictures, carcinoma, radiation cystitis, and urethral caruncles. In the male, urethroprostatitis can cause bleeding into the urine (James 1976). Vigorous exercise by normal individuals can result in hematuria (Fred and Natelson 1977), and Fred (1978) has concluded that this type of bleeding originates in the urinary bladder, but the mechanism for this occurrence is still only conjectural. Hematuria that is a result of exercise is only transitory.

Hematuria may be present in any bleeding disorder such as leukemia (Boyd 1977), thrombocytopenia, coagulation factor deficiencies, sickle cell disease or trait, and in scurvy which can be seen in malnourished individuals (Lytton 1977). Anticoagulant drugs may also cause hematuria. The use of penicillins and cephalosporins can cause an acute interstitial nephritis or a hemorrhagic cystitis which is manifested by hematuria (Chudwin et al. 1979, James 1976). Hematuria may accompany fever and subacute bacterial endocarditis, and may be the result of toxic reactions to various drugs. Studies by Freni et al. (1977) show that tobacco smoking causes raised levels of ortho-aminophenols as a result of abnormal tryptophan metabolism. These metabolites are known to be carcinogenic and may be the reason why the studies showed a significant relation between smoking and microhematuria. There have been some cases reported in which hematuria has resulted from the increased consumption of soda pop (Thompson 1978).

It should be remembered that hematuria in a female may be the result of menstrual contamination.

Hemoglobinuria

Hemoglobinuria is the presence of free hemoglobin in the urine as a result of intravascular hemolysis. The hemolysis that occurs in the urine while in the urinary tract or after voiding because of a low specific gravity or highly alkaline pH, may be considered to be hemoglobinuria, but it does not bear the same significance as true hemoglobinuria. Hemoglobinuria without hematuria occurs as a result of hemoglobinemia (free hemoglobin in the blood) and, therefore, it has primarily nothing to do with the kidneys even though it may secondarily result in kidney damage.

Normally, less than 10% of red cell destruction occurs intravascularly, the rest occurs in the reticuloendothelial (RE) cells (Hillman and Finch 1974). The hemoglobin that is released from the red cells quickly binds to a special plasma globulin called haptoglobin. The function of haptoglobin is to prevent the glomerular excretion of hemoglobin. This binding serves to conserve iron and to protect the tubules from the harmful effect of hemoglobin when some of it is reabsorbed (Hoffman 1970). The hemoglobin–haptoglobin complex is removed from the circulation by the RE system. The half-life of the hemoglobin–haptoglobin complex is 2–3 hours (Sisson 1976). Since during hemolysis haptoglobin is removed faster than it can be replaced, the plasma concentration will decrease; moreover, in severe hemolysis it can reach 0 level in 8–12 hours (Miale 1977).

Because haptoglobin binds hemoglobin stoichiometrically (1 mole to 1 mole), the concentration of haptoglobin determines the amount of hemoglobin that can be bound. Normal plasma levels of haptoglobin are about 100 mg/dl of plasma (Erslev and Gabuzda 1975, Ritchie 1979), so it is capable of binding hemoglobin to that same extent. Ritchie (1979) states that it is common for normal young adults to have steady-state haptoglobin values of 30–50 mg/dl, meaning that the destruction of 2 to 3.5 ml of red blood cells would remove all of the available haptoglobin. When the haptoglobin binding capacity is exceeded, hemoglobin will be lost in the urine. The free plasma hemoglobin, unattached to the high-molecular-weight haptoglobin, is readily filtered through the glomerulus. Some of the hemoglobin is reabsorbed into the tubular epithelial cells where its iron is removed and deposited within the cell as ferritin and hemosiderin. Hillman and Finch (1974) state that as much as 5 g/day of filtered hemoglobin can be processed without exceeding the tubular uptake capacity. The filtered hemoglobin which is not reabsorbed is lost in the urine. The presence of hemosiderin granules in tubular cells is a valuable sign that the patient either is suffering from intravascular hemolysis or has recently done so (see Chapter 5). When hemoglobin is filtered at the glomerulus, three things may happen: the excretion of only hemosiderin, of hemosiderin and hemoglobin, or of just hemoglobin if the hemolysis is acute and massive (Hillman and Finch 1974).

Some of the many conditions that are associated with intravascular hemolysis and which can therefore result in hemoglobinuria are: hemolytic anemias due to drugs, chemicals, and malarial parasites (blackwater fever); incompatible blood transfusions; severe burns; strenuous exercise such as marching (especially on hard pavement) and jogging; and, poisoning from snake venom, spider bites, and bacterial toxins. Hemoglobinuria can be found in severe diseases such as yellow fever and scarlet fever (Frankel 1963a). It can also be seen in paroxysmal nocturnal hemoglobinuria, and paroxysmal cold hemoglobinuria following exposure of all or part of the body to the cold. Sensitivity to the fava bean (favism) may result in severe hemolytic anemia. Hemolysis may also occur in individuals with a prosthetic heart valve.

The urine sample which contains hemoglobin may vary in color from normal to a dark brown (Coca-cola color) if acid, or pink to red if alkaline. Hemoglobinuria should be suspected when the test for occult blood is positive but the microscopic shows no RBCs, or if the degree of the positive test does not correspond to the number of RBCs in the microscopic. Myoglobinuria will show the same screening pattern as hemoglobinuria.

The presence of hemoglobin in the urine is always significant, however, it is not the hemoglobinuria that is important, but rather the intravascular hemolysis (Berman 1977).

Myoglobinuria

Myoglobin is the heme protein of striated muscle. It serves as a reserve supply of oxygen and also facilitates the movement of oxygen within muscle (Stryer 1975). Injury to cardiac or skeletal muscle results in the release of myoglobin into the circulation. Even just subtle injury to the muscle cells can bring about the release of myoglobin (Berman 1977). Myoglobin has a molecular weight of approximately 17,000 and so it is easily filtered through the glomerulus and excreted in the urine (Arnow 1966, Bauer et al. 1968, Sisson 1976). Since it is cleared so rapidly from the circulation, the plasma is left uncolored even though the urine may be red to brown to black, depending on the degree of myoglobinuria. Myoglobin is very toxic to the renal tubules and in large amounts it is associated with acute renal failure (Greenhill and Gruskin 1976, Bradley et al. 1979, Sisson 1976).

Myoglobinuria occurs with conditions involving destruction of muscle such as with crush injuries, severe or unaccustomed exercise, heat stroke, electric shock (Berman 1977), trauma including beatings, polymyositis, and convulsions. It can also be present with myocardial infarction (MI) and it has been suggested that screening for myoglobinuria may be useful as a clinical adjunct in the diagnosis of MI (Cloonan et al. 1976, Markowitz and Wobig 1977). Muscle is also destroyed in McArdle's disease, viral illnesses (Greenhill and Gruskin 1976), fish poisoning (Haff's disease), sea snake bites, hyperthermia, myositis due to trichinosis (Sisson 1976), infarction of large skeletal muscles, and in disorders associated with rhabdomyolysis, such as familial paroxysmal myoglobinuria.

Screening Tests

Those tests which screen for occult blood will detect hematuria, hemoglobinuria, and myoglobinuria. As previously mentioned, these states can coexist. If the correlation of the microscopic and chemical results does not imply hematuria, then further evaluation and studies may be done to determine the presence of hemoglobinuria vs. myoglobinuria. The definitive diagnostic test for differentiating these two states is electrophoresis (Sisson 1976). Other methods that can be used are immunodiffusion, hemagglutination inhibition, or immunoelectrophoresis.

Berman (1977) suggests the following guideline for a rapid differentiation of hemoglobinuria and myoglobinuria: red plasma plus red urine equals hemoglobin; clear plasma plus red urine equals myoglobin. Another screening procedure is the ammonium sulfate test which will be described in this section.

Testing for blood by using benzidine has long been the standard procedure for the detection of occult blood. Since benzidine has been found to be carcinogenic, the routine use of it has been discouraged, and so that procedure will not be included in this book.

REAGENT TEST-STRIPS

The dipstick procedure is based on the peroxidase-like activity of hemoglobin and myoglobin which catalyzes the oxidation of an indicator by an organic peroxide. In N-Multistix the indicator is 3,3',5,5'-tetramethylbenzidine and the peroxide is cumene hydroperoxide (Ames 1981). Chemstrip 8 uses the indicator tetramethylbenzidine and the peroxide is 2,5-dimethyl-2,5-dihydroperoxyhexane (Bio-Dynamics/bmc 1979a).

Both dipsticks are capable of detecting intact erythrocytes as well as free hemoglobin and myoglobin. Intact red blood cells in the urine will hemolyze on the test pad. The freed hemoglobin will react with the reagent and will result in green spots on a yellow or orange background. Thus, the presence of intact red cells will give a spotted green reaction, whereas free hemoglobin and myoglobin will give a uniform green or green to dark blue color.

N-Multistix is read at 25 seconds, and the color change is from orange to green to dark blue. It is generally capable of detecting 5 to 15 intact red cells per microliter, or 0.015 to 0.060 mg/dl of free hemoglobin (Ames 1981). The sensitivity is less in urines with high specific gravity or with an ascorbic acid content of more than 5 mg/dl. The test is slightly more sensitive to free hemoglobin and myoglobin than to intact red blood cells. The results are reported as trace through 3 + (or large). False-positive reactions may occur if the urine or test-strip is contaminated with Betadine (Rasoulpour et al. 1978).

Chemstrip 8 is read at 60 seconds and the color change is from yellow to green. The lowest concentration that can be detected is about 5 intact RBC/μl, or the amount of free hemoglobin equivalent to 10 RBC/μl. High levels of ascorbic acid will give lower test values or even false-negative results. The presence of nitrite in the urine in excess of 10 mg/dl will delay the test reaction (Bio-Dynamics/bmc 1979a). There are two separate color scales for erythrocytes and hemoglobin. The concentrations for the intact red cell color scale and the corresponding ranges are approximately 5–10 (5–15), 50 (30–100), and 250 RBC/μl (150–300). The concentrations for hemoglobin and the corresponding ranges are: 50 (30–150), and 250 RBC/μl (150–300) (BMC 1978).

Both dipsticks will give false-positive results in the presence of certain oxidizing contaminants such as hypochlorites which may be used to clean urine-collection containers. Studies by Smith et al. (1977) showed that sodium hypochlorite in the concentration of 100 mg/liter of urine gave a 2 + result with both dipsticks, which shows how sensitive the reagents are to oxidizing agents. When the urine is contaminated with a high bacterial content, a false-positive reaction may occur because of bacterial peroxidases (Wilson 1975). False positives will result if the urine is contaminated with menstrual blood.

Both dipsticks give lower or false-negative readings in the presence of high levels of ascorbic acid. If necessary, the test should be repeated at least 24 hours after the last dose of vitamin C. If the urine sample is not mixed well before testing, a false-negative result can occur because the red cells tend to settle in the bottom of the container.

HEMATEST

Hematest tablets (Ames Co.) can be used to test urine although they are usually used for detecting occult blood in stool specimens. The reagents in the tablet are: tartaric acid, calcium acetate, strontium peroxide, and the chromogen orthotolidine. When the Hematest tablet is moistened with water, the reagents are washed down onto the filter paper containing the sample. The tartaric acid and calcium acetate react with strontium peroxide to form hydrogen peroxide. The hemoglobin in the urine decomposes hydrogen peroxide with the liberation of oxygen, which then oxidizes orthotolidine to a blue-colored derivative.

This procedure is very insensitive when used for detecting occult blood in urine. It will not reliably detect less than 200 RBC/HPF (high power field) unless some of the cells have hemolyzed. It is more sensitive to free hemoglobin, detecting amounts produced by the hemolysis of 25–30 RBC/HPF (Ravel 1978).

PROCEDURE

1. Place 1 drop of urine on the filter paper.
2. Place a tablet in the center of the moistened portion of the filter paper.
3. Place 1 drop of water on top of the tablet, wait 5–10 seconds, then flow a second drop on the tablet so that it runs down the side and onto the filter paper.
4. If the test is positive, a blue color will appear on the filter paper around the tablet within 2 minutes. (The color of the tablet is of no significance.) The intensity of the color is proportional to the amount of red blood cells, hemoglobin, or myoglobin that is present, but it is difficult to try to semiquantitate the results. Report as positive or negative.

False-positive results: The contamination of the urine with hypochlorites or with large amounts of bacteria that have peroxidase activity can give false-positive results.

False-negative results: Because of the sensitivity of the procedure, urines containing less than 200 RBC/HPF or the hemoglobin contained in less than 25 RBC/HPF may appear as being negative for occult blood.

AMMONIUM SULFATE TEST
This procedure may be used to differentiate between hemoglobin-uria and myoglobinuria after a test for occult blood is positive, but few or no red cells are seen in the microscopic.

PROCEDURE. Prepare an 80% saturated urine solution of ammonium sulfate by adding 2.8 g of ammonium sulfate to 5 ml of urine in a test tube. Mix to dissolve. Filter or centrifuge. This procedure will precipitate out hemoglobin, but myoglobin will stay in solution. So if the supernatant is a normal color, then the precipitated pigment is hemoglobin; if the supernatant is colored, then the pigment is myoglobin.

Bilirubin and Urobilinogen

Bilirubin is formed from the breakdown of hemoglobin in the reticuloendothelial system. It is then bound to albumin and transported through the blood to the liver. This free or unconjugated bilirubin is insoluble in water and cannot be filtered through the glomerulus. In the liver, bilirubin is removed by the parenchymal cells and is conjugated with glucuronic acid to form bilirubin diglucuronide. This conjugated bilirubin, which is also called direct bilirubin, is water-soluble and is excreted by the liver through the bile duct and into the duodenum. Normally, very small amounts of conjugated bilirubin regurgitate back from the bile duct and into the blood system (Diggs 1971). Therefore, very small amounts of conjugated bilirubin can be found in the plasma, but not in concentrations higher than 0.2–0.4 mg/dl (Zimmerman 1979). Since conjugated bilirubin is not bound to protein, it is easily filtered through the glomerulus and excreted in the urine whenever the plasma level is increased. Normally, no detectable amount of bilirubin (sometimes referred to as "bile") can be found in the urine.

In the intestines, bacterial enzymes convert bilirubin through a group of intermediate compounds to several related compounds which are collectively referred to as "urobilinogen" (Zimmerman 1979). Most of the urobilinogen (a colorless pigment) and its oxidized variant, urobilin (a brown pigment), are lost in the feces. About 10 to 15% of the urobilinogen is reabsorbed into the bloodstream, returns to the liver, and is re-excreted into the intestines. A small amount of this urobilinogen is also excreted by the kidneys into the urine, with a normal level of about 1–4 mg/24 h or less than 1.0 Ehrlich unit/2 h (Sisson 1976, Zimmerman 1979). The diagram in Figure 2-1A demonstrates the normal pathway of bilirubin and uro-

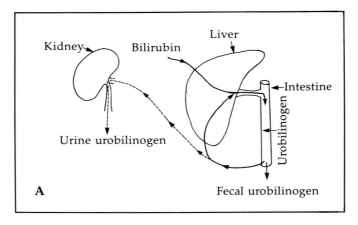

FIGURE 2-1A   **Normal pathway of bilirubin and urobilinogen.**

bilinogen. (The anatomical parts have been rearranged for the purpose of illustration.)

The normal level of total bilirubin in the serum is about 1.0 mg/dl or less (Krupp et al. 1979). This consists mainly of indirect or unconjugated bilirubin, but there is also a very small amount of direct or conjugated bilirubin present. When the level of total bilirubin exceeds approximately 2.5 mg/dl (Zimmerman 1979), the tissues of the body take on the yellow color of bilirubin, and this is called jaundice. If the jaundice is due to an increase in unconjugated bilirubin, no bilirubin will be excreted in the urine because unconjugated bilirubin cannot be filtered at the glomerulus. But if jaundice is due to an increase in the water-soluble conjugated bilirubin, then bilirubin will be present in the urine.

There are three major types of jaundice: hepatic, obstructive, and hemolytic. Since these types differ in the substances excreted in the urine, they can be differentiated by testing for the presence of bilirubin and urobilinogen.

The first type of jaundice to be discussed is that which results from liver damage. The clinical picture varies according to the type and degree of hepatic injury. There may be injury to the parenchymal cells caused by viral hepatitis or cirrhosis. Intrahepatic disease as a result of chemical intoxication or drug reactions can also cause hepatic jaundice. Figure 2-1B demonstrates the possible pathway in hepatic jaundice. The flow of conjugated bilirubin into the duodenum is inhibited, so the bilirubin backs up into the blood and jaundice may be present, depending on the degree of inhibition. In some types of liver damage, the liver may also not be able to conjugate the normal amount of bilirubin and so the resulting jaundice will be due to both conjugated and unconjugated bilirubin. Although there is partial obstruction to the flow of bilirubin into the duodenum, some

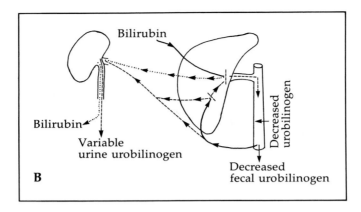

Bilirubin

Decreased
urobilinogen

Bilirubin

Variable
urine urobilinogen

Decreased
fecal urobilinogen

B

Pathway in hepatic jaundice.   **FIGURE 2-1B**

is still able to pass into the intestines where urobilinogen is formed. The feces will be lighter in color due to the decrease in urobilin, which is the oxidized form of urobilinogen. When part of the urobilinogen is reabsorbed, the liver may not be able to reabsorb or reexcrete the circulating urobilinogen, thus causing more to appear in the urine. The clinical picture in hepatic jaundice may be: positive urine bilirubin; decreased fecal urobilinogen; and, depending on the type of liver damage, either normal, decreased, or increased levels of urine urobilinogen.

In some kinds of liver cell damage, the normal pathway of bilirubin conjugation and excretion is not affected, but the liver cells are unable to remove the circulating urobilinogen. This can sometimes be seen in cirrhosis of the liver, metastatic carcinoma, and congestive heart failure (Zimmerman 1979). The resulting picture will then be: negative urine bilirubin, normal fecal urobilinogen, and increased urine urobilinogen.

The second major type of jaundice is obstructive jaundice, which may be due to an obstruction in the common bile duct caused by gallstones, carcinoma, pancreatitis, diseased lymph nodes surrounding the duct, or by carcinoma of the head of the pancreas. There may also be obstruction from intrahepatic blockage of small biliary ducts by tumors. Severe drug toxicity can also cause a type of intrahepatic obstruction (Ravel 1978). Figure 2-1C gives a good illustration of the path of bilirubin in the presence of total obstruction. The obstruction prevents the entry of bilirubin into the duodenum. The bilirubin backs up into the blood, which causes a jaundice due to conjugated bilirubin, and then bilirubin is excreted in the urine. Since bilirubin is unable to get into the intestines, urobilinogen cannot be formed; thus, the feces will have a characteristic "clay-colored" or gray-white appearance. The clinical picture in total obstruction is: positive urine bilirubin, negative urine urobilinogen, and negative

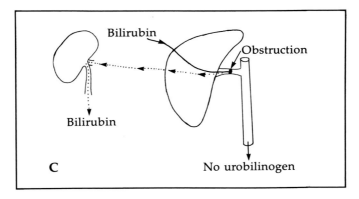

FIGURE 2-1C **Pathway in obstructive jaundice.**

or only very trace amounts of fecal urobilinogen. If the obstruction is only partial, then the clinical picture will resemble that which is seen in Figure 2-1*B*.

Hemolytic jaundice is that type of jaundice which is the result of the excessive production of bilirubin. The increased breakdown of red blood cells produces bilirubin at a rate that exceeds the ability of the liver to conjugate and excrete it. The jaundice is, therefore, due to unconjugated bilirubin. As shown in Figure 2-1*D*, the liver is able to excrete all of the conjugated bilirubin as it is formed, but the increased excretion of conjugated bilirubin results in an increased amount of fecal urobilinogen. This usually leads to more urobilinogen being reabsorbed from the intestines and, therefore, the urine will also contain increased levels. So the clinical picture in hemolytic jaundice is: negative urine bilirubin, increased urine urobilinogen, and increased fecal urobilinogen. In some cases there may also be a positive test for occult blood due to the presence of free he-

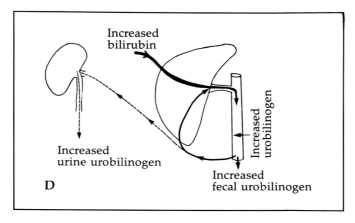

FIGURE 2-1D **Pathway in hemolytic jaundice.**

moglobin in the urine. Some of the possible causes of hemolytic jaundice include: intravascular hemolysis; anemia, especially hemolytic anemia; and thalassemia.

Screening Tests for Bilirubin (Bile)

The screening test for bilirubin is not necessarily part of the routine urinalysis in all laboratories. It is, however, frequently requested to be done when liver disease is suspected. Bilirubin can be detected in the urine before other clinical symptoms are present or recognizable. The detection of small quantities is very important in the early diagnosis of obstructive and hepatic jaundice (Assa 1977). This test is also useful in the differential diagnosis of obstructive (positive) and hemolytic (negative) jaundice.

Bilirubin is light sensitive and so the urine should be protected from the light and examined as quickly as possible. On standing and especially when exposed to light, bilirubin, which is a yellow-brown color, will be oxidized to biliverdin, which is a green color. Many of the procedures used to detect bilirubin will not react with biliverdin, so false-negative results may occur if the urine is not tested when fresh.

Detectable amounts of bilirubin are not normally present in the urine, so the results of some methods are just reported as positive or negative.

The procedure of choice when liver disease is suspected is the Ictotest, because of the sensitivity of the test.

REAGENT TEST-STRIPS

Both dipsticks are based on the coupling reaction of a diazonium salt with bilirubin in an acid medium. They differ, however, in the diazonium salt that is used and the color that develops.

N-Multistix contains 2,4-dichloroaniline diazonium salt. It is read at 20 seconds and the color change ranges from buff through various shades of tan or tannish-purple. The test has a sensitivity of 0.2−0.4 mg/dl of bilirubin.

Chemstrip 8 contains 2,6-dichlorobenzene-diazonium-tetrafluoroborate. It is read at 30−60 seconds, and the color changes from white to pink to red-violet depending on the bilirubin concentration. The test detects 0.5 mg/dl of bilirubin.

The results on both dipsticks can be reported as 1+ through 3+, or as small (slight), moderate, or large (strong). The color of the dipstick must be carefully compared with the color chart in order to get accurate results.

False-negative results: These can occur in the presence of large amounts of ascorbic acid, elevated concentrations of nitrite, or if the bilirubin has been oxidized to biliverdin.

False-positive results: Patients receiving large doses of chlorpromazine may have false-positive results. Metabolites of drugs such as phenazopyridine which give a red color at a low pH may also cause false positives.

ICTOTEST

The Ictotest (Ames Co.) is a tablet test that is based on the same diazo reaction as the dipsticks. It is, however, much more sensitive than the dipsticks, being able to detect as little as 0.05 to 0.1 mg/dl. Because of this sensitivity, Ictotest is the recommended procedure when a test for just bilirubin is ordered. It also serves as a good confirmatory test for a positive dipstick.

The tablet contains the following reagents: p-nitrobenzene-diazonium p-toluenesulfonate, sulfosalicylic acid, sodium bicarbonate, and boric acid. The mats that are used in the procedure are made of an asbestos—cellulose mixture. When the urine is placed on the mat, the absorbent qualities of the mat cause the bilirubin to remain on the outer surface. The sulfosalicylic acid provides the acid environment for the reaction. It also acts with the sodium bicarbonate to provide an effervescence which helps to partially dissolve the tablet. The diazonium salt then couples with the bilirubin on the mat, giving a blue or purple reaction product.

PROCEDURE

1. Place 5 drops of urine on one square of the special test mat supplied with Ictotest.
2. Place a tablet in the center of the moistened area.
3. Flow 2 drops of water onto the tablet so that the water runs off of the tablet and onto the mat.
4. Observe the color of the mat around the tablet at the end of 30 seconds. If a blue or purple color develops, the test is positive. All other colors including pink or red are negative.

False-positive results: Urine from patients receiving large doses of chlorpromazine (Thorazine) may give false-positive reactions.

If the urine is suspected of containing a large amount of chlorpromazine, the wash-through technique can be used. Prepare duplicate mats with 5 drops of urine on each. To one mat add 10 drops of water to wash through the drug metabolites. Add a tablet to each mat and perform the Ictotest procedure. If the color is about the same on both mats, bilirubin is present, since it stays adsorbed on the mat surface. If the wash-through mat is either much lighter or if no color is present, then the reaction is probably due to the drug metabolites (Free and Free 1978).

FOAM TEST

If the urine is a yellowish-brown or greenish-yellow color and bilirubin is suspected, shake the urine. If a yellow or greenish-yellow foam develops, then bilirubin is most likely present. Bilirubin alters the surface tension of urine and foam will develop after shaking. The yellow color is from the bilirubin pigment. A false-positive test will be given when the urine contains phenazopyridine (Lippman 1957).

The foam test must be followed up by another more accurate procedure. It can, however, be a good clue that bilirubin is present, and the technologist should then test out the possibility of bilirubinuria.

SMITH IODINE TEST
Place 5 ml of acid urine in a test tube. Overlay the urine with 2 ml of 0.7% iodine in 95% ethyl alcohol. When bile is present, an emerald-green ring will develop at the junction of the two liquids. The test is sensitive to 0.3–1 mg/dl of bilirubin (Henry 1964). Report the results as positive or negative.

HARRISON SPOT TEST
In the Harrison spot test, barium chloride combines with sulfate radicals in the urine forming a precipitate of barium sulfate. Any bile pigments present will adhere to these large molecules. Ferric chloride in the presence of trichloroacetic acid will then oxidize yellow bilirubin to green biliverdin (Baker et al. 1966). This procedure is very sensitive and is said to detect 0.005–0.1 mg/dl of bilirubin (Henry 1964).

REAGENTS
1. Fouchet's reagent—Combine the following:
    Trichloroacetic acid—25 g
    10% ferric chloride solution—10 ml
    Distilled water—100 ml
2. 10% barium chloride solution

PROCEDURE
1. Add 5 ml of 10% barium chloride solution to 10 ml of acidified urine.
2. Shake well and filter to remove the precipitate.
3. Spread the precipitate out on another filter paper and allow to dry.
4. Add 1 drop of Fouchet's reagent to the precipitate. If bilirubin is present, a green or blue-green color will develop. Report as positive or negative.

Barium chloride-impregnated strips of heavy filter paper can also be used. Moisten a strip of barium chloride paper with urine and add one drop of Fouchet's reagent to the wet area.

Screening Tests for Urobilinogen
Testing for urobilinogen is not usually part of a routine urinalysis unless the laboratory uses the 7 or 8 multiple dipstick. However, it is

a useful screening test in the diagnosis of liver function and, as such, it is frequently requested to be performed on urine.

There are two other factors other than liver disease which must be taken into account when interpreting a urobilinogen result. Patients receiving broad-spectrum antibiotics and other substances which will alter the normal bacterial flora in the intestines, will excrete little or no urobilinogen in their urine because urobilinogen cannot be formed in the intestines. Also, in cases of intestinal obstruction, significant quantities of urobilinogen may be absorbed from the intestine and thus the urine levels will increase (Sobotka et al. 1953).

Unlike bilirubin, urobilinogen is normally present in the urine but in concentrations of 1 Ehrlich unit or less per 100 ml of urine. Some of the procedures will only detect amounts in excess of this, but the dipsticks are capable of detecting normal amounts. Decreased or absent levels of urobilinogen cannot be detected by any of these screening procedures.

One of the important problems in measuring urobilinogen is its instability. The urobilinogen is converted to urobilin on standing in the presence of oxygen and on exposure to air. For this reason, the test should be performed on a fresh specimen.

Urobilinogen excretion seems to be at its peak level between 2 and 4 p.m., so when screening for liver damage it is advisable to do a collection during these hours (Simmons and Gentskow 1955, Alba 1975, Bauer et al. 1968).

The following procedures are qualitative. There are, however, several quantitative methods available for the detection of urobilinogen. Chapter 5 includes a qualitative procedure known as the Watson-Schwartz test which can be used to differentiate urobilinogen and porphobilinogen.

REAGENT TEST-STRIPS

Each brand of dipstick involves a different reaction.

N-Multistix is based on the Ehrlich aldehyde reaction. The reagent is *p*-dimethylaminobenzaldehyde which reacts with urobilinogen in a strongly acid medium to produce a color change from yellow to a brown-orange. It is capable of detecting concentrations as low as 0.1 Ehrlich U/dl. There are two normal blocks on the color chart for 0.1 and 1 Ehrlich U/dl and these can either be reported as "normal", or by giving the numerical value. The other color blocks are for 2, 4, 8, and 12 Ehrlich units, and intermediary values may be estimated by interpolation between the blocks. The color is read at 45 seconds.

N-Multistix is not specific for urobilinogen. Porphobilinogen, indole, and skatole will give the same color development as urobilinogen. There is minimal interference by pigments such as bilirubin and hemoglobin. However, there are other substances which can interfere with this procedure, such as sulfisoxazole, p-aminosalicylic acid, and phenazopyridine, but they give an atypical color reaction (Hager and Free 1970).

Chemstrip 8 contains the reagent 4-methoxybenzene-diazonium-tetrafluoroborate which reacts with urobilinogen in an acid medium to produce a red azo dye. Thus, the color change is from white through pink to orange-red. The color reaction is almost instantaneous, and its intensity is an index of urobilinogen concentration. Values can be read at 10 to 30 seconds. The lowest limit of detection is about 0.4 mg/dl, and the results may be reported the same way as with N-Multistix.

Nitrite concentrations above 5 mg/dl, and formalin concentrations above 200 mg/dl may cause a decrease in the color reaction of Chemstrip 8 (Bio-Dynamics/bmc 1979a). Urine from patients receiving phenazopyridine may show a false-positive reaction.

EHRLICH'S QUALITATIVE TEST
Before the introduction of the dipstick procedure, Ehrlich's test was the standard qualitative screening test.

EHRLICH'S REAGENT
p-dimethylaminobenzaldehyde—10 g
Concentrated HCl—75 ml
Distilled water—75 ml

PROCEDURE
1. Place 10 ml of freshly voided urine in a test tube and allow it to reach room temperature.
2. Add 1 ml of Ehrlich's reagent and mix.
3. Let stand for 5 minutes.
4. Normal amounts of urobilinogen will change the solution to a pink color which can be observed by looking down through the tube. High levels of urobilinogen will give a cherry-red color.

Porphobilinogen is also detected by this method. The addition of 5 ml of saturated sodium acetate solution (150 g of anhydrous sodium acetate plus 100 ml of water) will intensify the color if due to urobilinogen but not if due to the presence of porphobilinogen (Baker et al. 1966). Phenazopyridine, indole, and p-aminosalicylic acid will also yield a pink to red color which is indistinguishable from that produced by urobilinogen.

This test may be used as a semiquantitative procedure by diluting the urine 1:10, 1:20, 1:30, 1:40 etc. Report the highest dilution which shows the slightest pink color (Frankel 1963a). Color reactions are normal in dilutions up to 1:20 (Krupp et al. 1979).

Nitrite

The nitrite test is a rapid, indirect method for the early detection of significant and asymptomatic bacteriuria. Common organisms which can cause urinary tract infections, such as *Escherichia coli, Enterobacter, Citrobacter, Klebsiella,* and *Proteus* species, contain enzymes which reduce the nitrate in the urine to nitrite. For this to occur, the urine must have incubated in the bladder for a minimum of four hours. Hence, the first morning urine is the specimen of choice.

The urine should be tested shortly after being voided, because if the urine is allowed to stand at room temperature for several hours, organisms may grow in the specimen and generate nitrite (Free and Free 1978).

A negative test should never be interpreted as indicating the absence of bacterial infection. There are several reasons for this: 1) there may be pathogens present in the urine that do not form nitrite; 2) the urine may not have remained in the bladder long enough for the nitrate to be converted to nitrite; 3) there are cases in which the urine does not contain any nitrate, so bacteria may be present but the dipstick will be negative; and 4) under certain circumstances, the bacterial enzymes may have reduced nitrate to nitrite and then converted nitrite to nitrogen, which will give a negative nitrite result (Ames 1976). Studies by James et al. (1978c) have shown that false-negative nitrite determinations or negative interferences can be the result of abnormally high levels of urobilinogen, the presence of ascorbic acid levels as low as 5 mg/dl, and when the urinary pH is 6.0 or less.

The nitrite test is not meant to take the place of other routine bacteriology studies such as cultures and smears. The dipstick procedure is just used as a screening test which is capable of detecting bacteriuria even when not clinically suspected. If there are clinical symptoms, then regular bacteriology tests should be performed, even if the nitrite test is negative. There are other rapid nitrite tests that can be done in the bacteriology lab to give the physician temporary information until the cultures have time to grow. These include Microstix (Ames Co.) (Gatenby et al. 1974) and Bac-U-Dip (Warner–Chilcott Laboratories) (Randolph and Morris 1974). Since these dipsticks are not used for the routine urinalysis, they will not be discussed here.

N-Multistix

At the acid pH of the reagent area, nitrite reacts with *p*-arsanilic acid to form a diazonium compound. This compound then couples with 1, 2, 3, 4-tetrahydro-benzo(h)quinolin-3-ol to produce a pink color. The strip is read at 40 seconds. Any degree of uniform pink color should be interpreted as a positive nitrite test suggesting the presence of 10^5 or more organisms per ml. The color development is not proportional to the number of bacteria present. Pink spots or pink edges should not be considered a positive result. If the uniform pink color is very light, it may best be seen by placing the strip against a white paper.

This test has a sensitivity of 0.03–0.06 mg/dl of nitrite ion in urines of normal specific gravity and moderate levels of ascorbic acid (less than 25 mg/dl). The sensitivity of the test is reduced in urine with a high specific gravity or elevated level of ascorbic acid, as well as in the previously discussed reasons. The test is reported as positive or negative.

Chemstrip 8

In the Chemstrip 8 method, an aromatic amine, sulfanilamide, reacts with nitrite in the presence of an acid buffer to produce a diazonium salt. This diazonium salt then couples with 3-hydroxy-1,2,3,4-tetra-hydrobenz-(h)-quinoline, forming an azo dye. The intensity of the red color reflects the concentration of nitrite present, but does not constitute an index of the severity of the infection (BMC 1978). The test is read at 30 seconds, and the color change is from white to pale pink to red.

It is possible to detect concentrations of only 0.05 mg/dl with a pale pink coloration. Treatment with drugs containing phenazo-pyridine may cause a color reaction that is somewhat similar to that of a positive nitrite test. The sensitivity of the test is decreased in the presence of large amounts of ascorbic acid.

Quality Control and Instrumentation

Quality control should play an important part in the routine urinalysis laboratory. Because of the subjective nature of many of the tests performed in this section of the laboratory (e.g., visual interpretation of dipsticks, microscopic examination), it is rather difficult to implement a rigid quality control (Q.C.) program. However, it is because of the subjectivity of these procedures that a good Q.C. program must be established.

Urine controls should be run to monitor the reagent strip tests and all of the other qualitative chemical procedures. There are several commercial controls available for monitoring the dipstick and specific gravity tests, or some labs may prefer to make their own composite controls. Various recipes for composite controls can be found in Bradley et al. (1979), Ottaviano and DiSalvo (1977), and McNeely (1980). When possible, all qualitative tests should be run with both positive and negative controls. Positive controls for these procedures may be either contrived samples or preserved specimens from known positive samples.

A routine urinalysis quality control program should incorporate the following points:

1. The procedure manual should give a detailed description of each procedure, list which confirmatory tests should be used for positive results, and describe which controls are to be used with each test.
2. Positive and negative controls should be run at least once a shift. Where possible, introduce split specimens as "hidden" controls. Record results of the controls and ascertain if an "in-control" situation is occurring.
3. Record temperatures of refrigerators, water baths, and, where applicable, osmometers.
4. Daily, calibrate and run controls on any instrument, such as the refractometer or osmometer.
5. Do preventative maintenance on instruments (i.e., microscope, centrifuge, automated and semi-automated instruments).
6. Follow manufacturer's directions for storage and use of reagent strips. Compare dipstick results carefully with the color chart provided.
7. When preparing the urinary sediment, use a specific amount as well as a definite speed and time for centrifugation. Some controls are now available for the microscopic test.

In an effort to remove some of the subjectivity from the routine urinalysis, both dipstick manufacturers now offer a semi-automated instrument for reading their respective reagent strips. The use of an instrument for reading the hand-dipped reagent strips eliminates errors involving variations in operator timing and technique, differences in the perception of color among personnel, and differences in lighting conditions. Both the Clini-Tek from Ames Company and the Urotron from the Boehringer Mannheim Corporation can read up to eight different test results. These include pH, protein, glucose, ketones, bilirubin, occult blood, urobilinogen, and nitrite. Both machines are based on the principle of reflectance, with the amount of light reflected being inversely related to the concentration of substances present.

The Clini-Tek uses specially designed reagent strips which contain a white reference block with which the instrument identifies the type of strip to be read. The test results appear on a readout display panel on the front of the instrument, and an optional printer can be obtained to provide a written record of the results. The instrument may also be interfaced with a computer. Refer to Peele et al. (1977a and 1977b) for the results of a study on the comparison of visual vs. reflectance reading and an evaluation of reproducibility on the Clini-Tek.

The Urotron is programmed as to which type of strip is being used by the insertion of a coding card. The specially designed reagent strips contain an extra blank patch that is used for subtracting the color of the individual urine, thus eliminating interference from urinary color. The results are recorded on a chart recorder and the instrument can be interfaced with a computer.

The Clinilab (Ames Co.) is an automated instrument which performs seven chemical tests (i.e., pH, protein, glucose, ketones, bilirubin, occult blood, and urobilinogen) as well as the specific gravity of urine. The chemical tests are similar to those on the reagent strips. The specific gravity is measured by the falling drop method, in which the specific gravity is related to the time it takes for a drop of urine to pass between two sets of photo cells. A high specific gravity specimen is heavier and falls more quickly than does a dilute specimen.

Highly pigmented urine specimens can give false-positive chemical results if the urinary color is within the color-transmission band of the respective test filter (Clemens and Hurtle 1972). For this reason, highly colored urines should be tested by hand.

The Clinilab is capable of handling 120 specimens per hour and can, therefore, be useful in a high volume laboratory. This instrument can be interfaced with a computer system.

3

Microscopic Examination of the Urinary Sediment

The microscopic examination is a vital part of the routine urinalysis. It is a valuable diagnostic tool for the detection and evaluation of renal and urinary tract disorders as well as other systemic diseases. The value of the microscopic examination is dependent on two main factors: the examination of a suitable specimen, and the knowledge of the person performing the examination.

The best specimen for the routine urinalysis is the first morning specimen. Casts and red blood cells tend to dissolve or lyse in specimens with a low specific gravity or alkaline pH. The first morning specimen usually provides the concentrated and acidic environment needed to maintain these structures. The sediment should be examined as soon as possible after collection, but it may be refrigerated for a few hours if the examination cannot be performed immediately.

There have been some advances made in an effort to aid the technologist with the microscopic examination. These include the use of stains and the development of the phase and interference contrast microscopy techniques.

The most common stain for urinary sediments is the Sternheimer-Malbin supravital stain (Sternheimer and Malbin 1951, Sternheimer 1975, Abbott 1961). It contains crystal violet and safranin stains, and can be used as a general stain for most urinary structures. Some of the other staining techniques which can be used to differentiate certain urinary components include: Sudan III, Sudan IV, and Oil Red O, which are used to stain fat a pink to red color; eosin, which stains RBCs and helps to distinguish them from yeast cells which will not pick up the stain; and iodine, which can be used to stain starch granules and vegetable fibers a dark brown. These staining techniques will not be discussed here, because the aim of this book is to familiarize the reader with the appearance of unstained urinary sediment structures viewed with the brightfield microscope. Individuals who wish to routinely use sediment stains are referred to one of the previously mentioned references for the Sternheimer-Malbin stain.

The phase contrast microscope and the interference contrast microscope are both relatively new instruments for the study of unstained sediment material. Phase and interference contrast microscopy make transparent objects visible by changing the amplitude of light waves as they pass through the objects. Phase microscopy artificially retards diffracted light by one-fourth of a wavelength, and this produces a halo where the surfaces of slightly differing refractile indices meet one another. The interference contrast microscope produces its image by the splitting of light into two distinct beams. One beam passes through the object while the other serves as a reference. The beams are then recombined before being received, and this gives the object a relief or "three-dimensional" appearance. Brody et al. (1971) feel that phase microscopy should be used for the routine microscopic examination of urine. Haber (1972) states that interference contrast microscopy is useful in teaching morphologic identification of structures in the urinary sediment.

Although both phase and interference contrast techniques can be useful in the identification of urinary structures, in practice, few laboratories can afford the microscopes which are capable of being adapted for these techniques. This chapter will, therefore, present material which will help the technologist to become proficient at identifying the unstained specimen with the brightfield microscope. There are two microscopic techniques which will also be mentioned here. First, the use of polarized light for the identification of fat and other anisotropic substances. This can be done by the use of two polarizing filters, one is placed in the condenser and the other is placed on the ocular. The field is then darkened by rotating one of the filters (this crosses the polarizing filters at 90°) (Kurtzman and Rogers 1974). Secondly, colored filters can be placed below the condenser to help bring out the details of some structures. Filters can be very helpful when trying to photograph objects such as hyaline casts, which tend to blend in with the background.

The photomicrographs in this book include not only the abnormal structures found in the urine, but also those elements which have no pathological significance. The author feels that it is important to be able to recognize all structures found in the urine, otherwise, if one is not familiar with routine structures, then one will not be able to recognize something as being abnormal. The magnification given for the photomicrographs is approximately the magnification of the print itself. The value of the photomicrograph is limited in that only one focal plane can be seen, whereas in practice, the individual is able to see what is on all planes by constantly focusing up and down.

Preparation of the Sediment and use of the Microscope

The microscopic examination should be performed on a centrifuged sample. (If the volume of the specimen is too small to be centrifuged [i.e., just a few drops], then examine the sample directly, but note in the report that the results are from an uncentrifuged urine.) Mix the specimen and then place approximately 10–15 ml of urine into a centrifuge tube, and centrifuge at 2000 rpm for about 5 minutes. In an attempt to standardize the microscopic examination, the laboratory should adopt a regulated speed, time, and amount for the centrifugation of the urine specimens. Pour off the supernatant fluid (this can be used for confirmatory protein testing), and resuspend the sediment in the urine that drains back down from the sides of the tube. (Some labs leave exactly 1 ml of sediment and supernatant in the tube.) Flick the bottom of the tube to mix the sediment, and place a drop of sediment on a clean slide or in a counting chamber. Cover with a coverslip and examine immediately.

The first rule for examining unstained urinary sediment with the brightfield microscope is that subdued light *must* be used to provide adequate contrast. This is obtained by partially closing the iris diaphragm and then adjusting the condenser downward until optimum contrast is achieved. If there is too much light, some of the structures will be missed. For example, hyaline casts, which are gelled protein, have a very low refractive index and will be overlooked if the light is too bright or if there is not enough contrast.

The second important rule is that the fine adjustment should be continuously adjusted up and down to enable the viewer to see the depth of the object as well as other structures which may be on a different focal plane. Figure 3-1A is an example of why the focus should be constantly adjusted. The field seems to contain only amorphous phosphates (pH is 7.5); but, when the fine adjustment knob is moved slightly, look what else shows up in Figure 3-1B, a hyaline cylindroid!

The sediment should be viewed first under low power magnification (100×). Scan the slide and observe for casts, crystals, and elements that are present in only a few fields. Switch to high dry power (400×) when necessary to delineate the structures that are seen. Casts have a tendency to move towards the edge of the coverslip, so the entire periphery of the coverslip should be scanned. Some technologists prefer to first view the sediment under low

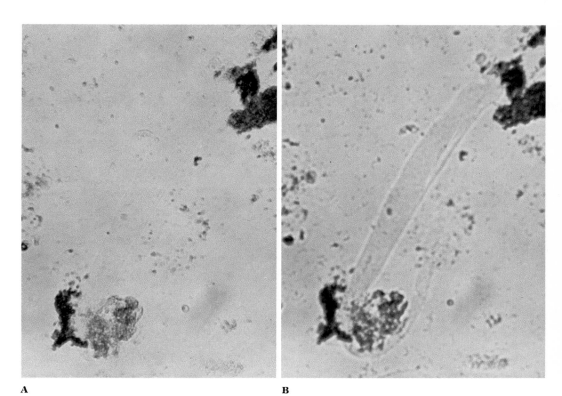

A   B

Amorphous phosphates and hyaline cylindroid. The   FIGURE 3-1
cylindroid is not visible in A, but appears in B when the
focus is adjusted. (200×).

power and without a coverslip. In this way they can observe for casts
in a concentrated area and without having them pushed towards the
edge of the coverslip. A coverslip is then applied and the sediment is
screened for other structures. While scanning under low power,
casts, crystals, and other elements can be noted and reported according to type as well as by giving an estimation of their number. Casts
can be reported as the average number that is present in 10–15 fields
under low power magnification (100×). For example, if the number
of hyaline casts in 10 different fields is: 1, 3, 2, 1, 1, 2, 2, 3, 1, and 3,
then the report would be: 1–3 hyaline casts/LPF. Some laboratories
prefer to report casts, epithelial cells, and structures other than WBCs
and RBCs, as "rare", "few", "moderate", "many", and "numerous".

Crystals need only be reported as being present, unless they are very abundant. Red blood cells, white blood cells, and epithelial cells are counted under high power (400×), and the average number in 10–15 fields is reported (e.g., 20–25 RBC/HPF).

Cells

The cells which can be present in the urine include erythrocytes (red blood cells or RBCs), leukocytes (white blood cells or WBCs), and epithelial cells from anywhere in the urinary tract from the tubules to the urethra or as contaminants from the vagina or vulva.

Erythrocytes

The red cells in the urine may have originated in any part of the urinary tract from the glomerulus to the urethral meatus, and in the female they may be the result of menstrual contamination. They can appear in a variety of forms depending upon the environment of the urine (Fig. 3-2). When the urine specimen is fresh, the red cells have a normal, pale, or yellowish appearance, and are smooth, biconcave disks approximately 7μ in diameter and 2μ thick. They contain no nuclei and, when viewed from the side, they have an hourglass appearance. In dilute or hypotonic urine, the red cells swell up and can lyse, thus releasing their hemoglobin into the urine. Lysed cells, which are referred to as "ghost" or "shadow" cells, are faint, colorless circles and are actually the empty red cell membranes. Lysing will also occur in alkaline urine. In hypertonic urine the red cells will crenate, and sometimes the crenations may resemble granules. Occasionally, small microcytic red cells can be seen in the urine sediment.

There are some structures that can be confused with red cells in the microscopic examination. When the red cells are swollen or crenated, they can sometimes be mistaken for WBCs. This is especially true if there is only one type of cell present in the sediment and so comparisons cannot be made between the cells. White cells are larger than red cells and they contain nuclei and are usually granular. But if the urine is hypotonic and the red cells have swollen, then it is possible to have problems differentiating the type of cell that is present. The presence of a positive test for occult blood is often helpful in making a decision. The author has found another useful hint in helping to decide if the cells are red cells or white cells. In Figure 3-3A, which shows a field with both red cells and white cells, there should not be any problem differentiating the two types of cells. The red cells in the figure resemble those that are seen in a blood smear; one can even see the hemoglobin in them. Now, by turning the fine

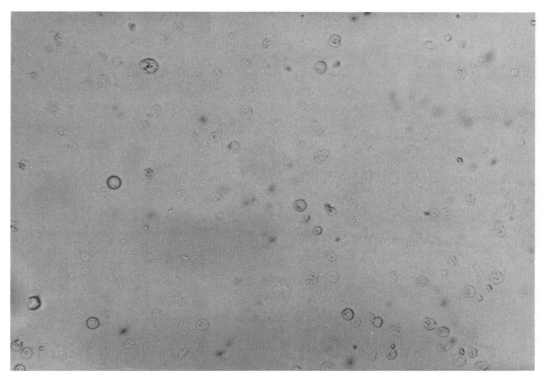

Red blood cells. The field also contains a white cell and several "ghost" cells. (400 ×).

FIGURE 3-2

adjustment up and down, the result is that the red cells "pop out" at the viewer as black circles, and this is seen is Figure 3-3*B*. The reason for this occurrence is that the red cells are very refractile and are thicker on the edges than in the center. This phenomenon will not occur if the red cells are grossly distorted by a hypotonic or hypertonic urine environment. The best way to differentiate red cells is by the addition of a few drops of 2% acetic acid. The red cells will lyse in dilute acetic acid, but white cells will not. The addition of the acid will also emphasize the nuclei of the WBCs. Since the acid will lyse the red cells, it is important to count the cells that are present before adding the acid. It is also advisable to scan the entire slide before the acid is added, otherwise, structures such as red cell casts will also dissolve, or new crystals will precipitate out.

Yeast cells can be mistaken for RBCs. Yeast cells are ovoid, rather than round, and they frequently contain buds which are smaller than themselves in size. The doubly refractile border of the

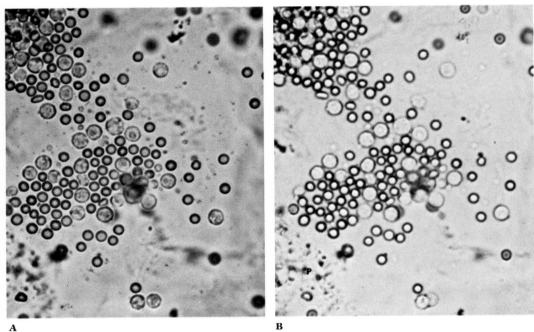

A   B

FIGURE 3-3   **RBCs and WBCs.** Changing the focus causes the red cells to
appear as black circles. (400 ×).

yeast cell tends to resemble the doughnut appearance of the red cell.
Yeast cells will not dissolve in 2% acetic acid, nor will they stain with
eosin.

Normally, red cells do not appear in the urine, although the
presence of 1–2 RBC/HPF is usually not considered abnormal (Wilson 1975, Bradley et al. 1979, ROCOM 1975, Hoffman 1970). The
mechanism whereby red cells enter the urine is not entirely clear
(Lippman 1957). Unlike white cells, red cells do not possess ameboid
characteristics and, therefore, they must stay within the blood vessels. Injury or rupture of the blood vessels of the kidney or urinary
tract releases red cells into the urine, but this does not account for the
acceptance of the normal presence of a few RBCs in the urine.

Hematuria is the presence of an increased number of RBCs in
the urine and the causes of hematuria are discussed in Chapter 2. If
large amounts of blood are present, the plasma protein will give a
positive protein test. As always, a correlation should be made be-

tween the chemical tests and the results of the microscopic examination.

Leukocytes

White cells can enter the urinary tract anywhere from the glomerulus to the urethra. On the average, the normal urine can contain up to 2 WBC/HPF (Baker et al. 1966, Wright 1959, Greenhill and Gruskin 1976). The white cells are approximately $10-12\mu$ in diameter (Race and White 1979) and are, therefore, larger than red cells but smaller than renal epithelial cells. White cells are usually spherical, and can appear as a dull gray or as a greenish-yellow color (Fig. 3-4). They may occur singly or in clumps (Fig. 3-5). The white cells in the urine are mostly neutrophils and they can usually be identified by their characteristic granules or by the lobulations of the nucleus. Figure 3-6 shows a field that is loaded with WBCs. The addition of 2% acetic acid to the slide accentuated the nuclei of the cells.

White blood cells in a hypotonic urine. The nuclei and granules are easily recognized. (800 ×).

FIGURE 3-4

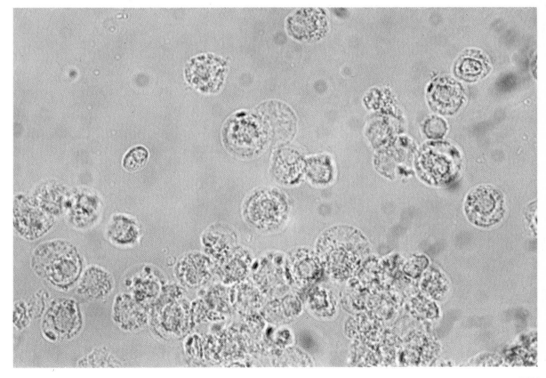

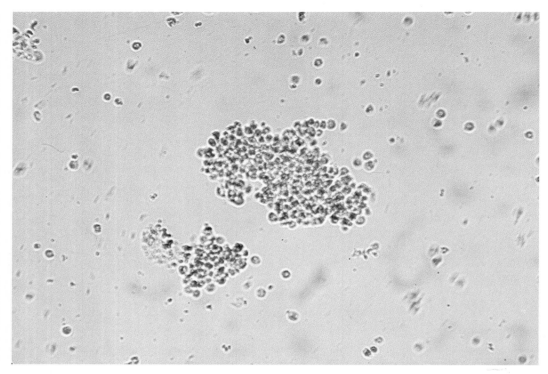

FIGURE 3-5   **White cell clumps.** (200 ×).

Leukocytes shrink in hypertonic urine, and swell up or are rapidly lysed in hypotonic or alkaline urine. Studies by Triger and Smith (1966) show that in an alkaline and hypotonic urine, the number of white cells decreases by 50% within an hour after collection if kept at room temperature. At 4°C, a 50% reduction will occur in two and a half hours.

When white cells expand in a dilute or hypotonic urine, their granules may demonstrate brownian movement. Cells which develop this characteristic are called "glitter cells". These glitter cells were formerly considered to be specific for pyelonephritis, but it is now understood that they can occur in a variety of conditions if the cells are exposed to a hypotonic environment (Berman et al. 1956).

An increase in WBCs in the urine is associated with an inflammatory process in or adjacent to the urinary tract. Leukocytes are attracted to any area of inflammation and, because of their ameboid properties, they can penetrate the areas adjacent to the inflammatory site. Sometimes pyuria (pus in the urine) is seen in conditions such as appendicitis and pancreatitis (Race and White 1979). It is also found in noninfectious conditions such as acute glomerulonephritis,

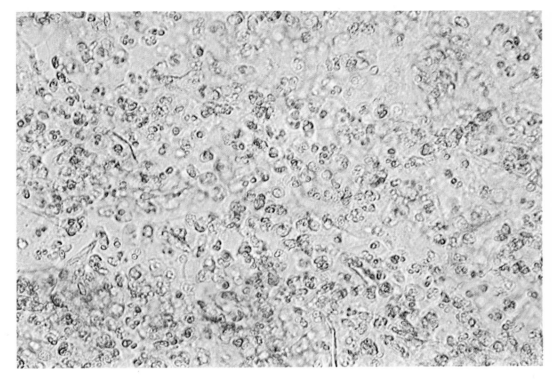

Numerous white cells.   Acetic acid (2%) was added to accentuate the nuclei. (400×).   FIGURE 3-6

lupus nephritis, renal tubular acidosis, dehydration, stress, fever, and in noninfectious irritation to the ureter, bladder, or urethra. The presence of many white cells in the urine, especially when they are in clumps, is strongly suggestive of acute infection such as pyelonephritis, cystitis, or urethritis (Weller 1971). White cell casts are evidence that the white cells are originating in the kidney. White cell clumps are also strongly suggestive of renal origin, but they are not conclusive evidence (Ravel 1978). Because of the importance of white cell clumps, their presence should be reported.

A few leukocytes can normally be found in secretions from the male and female genital tracts, so the possibility of a contaminated urine should be considered (Bradley et al. 1979).

Epithelial Cells

The epithelial cells in the urine may originate from any site in the genitourinary tract from the proximal convoluted tubule to the urethra, or from the vagina. Normally, a few cells from these sites can be found in the urine as a result of the normal sloughing off of old cells.

A marked increase indicates inflammation of that portion of the urinary tract from which the cells are derived.

It is very difficult to make a distinction between the epithelial cells that arise in the various portions of the urinary tract (Lippman 1957). For this reason, many laboratories report the presence of epithelial cells without attempting to differentiate them. When distinction is possible, three main types of epithelial cells may be recognized: tubular, transitional, and squamous.

RENAL TUBULAR EPITHELIAL CELLS

Renal tubular cells are slightly larger than leukocytes and contain a large round nucleus. They may be flat, cuboidal, or columnar. Figure 3-7 shows a field containing both white cells and tubular epithelial cells and demonstrates the difference in appearance between the two types of cells.

Increased numbers of tubular epithelial cells suggest tubular damage. This damage can occur in pyelonephritis, acute tubular necrosis, salicylate intoxication, and kidney transplant rejection.

FIGURE 3-7 **Renal epithelial cells (*arrow*) and numerous white cells.**
Note the size of the nucleus in each epithelial cell. (200×).

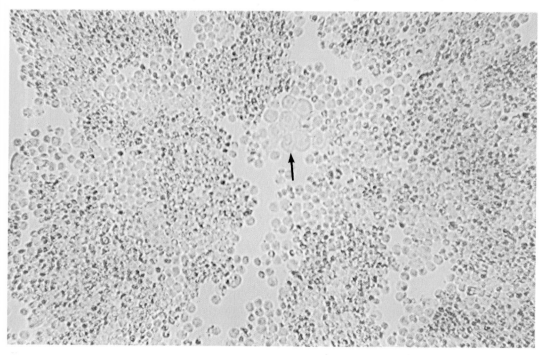

TRANSITIONAL EPITHELIAL CELLS

Transitional cells are two to four times as large as white cells. They may be round, pear-shaped, or may have tail-like projections. Occasionally these cells may contain two nuclei. Transitional cells line the urinary tract from the pelvis of the kidney to the upper portion of the urethra.

Figure 3-8 shows pear-shaped transitional cells, while Figure 3-9 demonstrates the size of a transitional cell in proportion to the size of white blood cells.

SQUAMOUS EPITHELIAL CELLS

Squamous epithelial cells are easily recognized as large, flat, irregularly-shaped cells. They contain small central nuclei and abundant cytoplasm (Fig. 3-10). The cell edge is often folded over and the cell may be rolled up into a cylinder. Squamous epithelial cells occur principally in the urethra and vagina. Many of the squamous cells present in the female urine are the result of contamination from the vagina or vulva, and as such, they have little diagnostic significance (Bradley et al. 1979).

Transitional epithelial cells. (500 ×). **FIGURE 3-8**

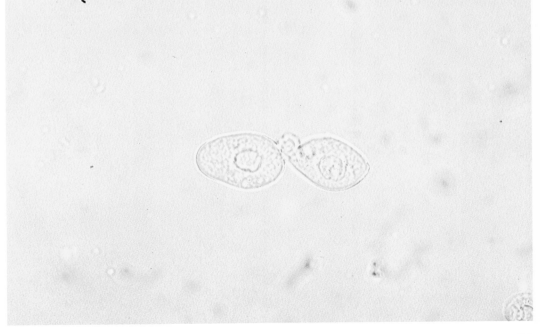

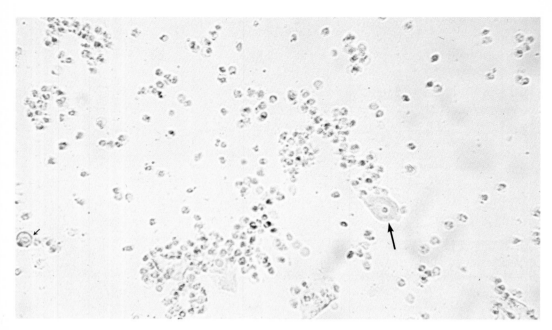

FIGURE 3-9   **Transitional epithelial cell (*large arrow*), several squamous epithelial cells and white cells.** Note the renal epithelial cell (*small arrow*). (200×).

FIGURE 3-10   **Squamous epithelial cells.** (160×).

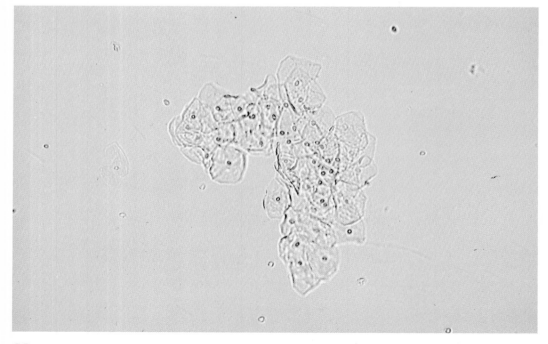

Crystals

Crystals are usually not found in freshly voided urine but appear after the urine stands for awhile. When the urine is supersaturated with a particular crystalline compound, or when the solubility properties of that compound are altered, the result is crystal formation. In some cases this precipitation occurs in the kidney or urinary tract, and can result in the formation of urinary calculi (stones).

Many of the crystals that are found in the urine have little clinical significance, except in cases of metabolic disorders, calculus formation, and the regulation of medication. The most important crystals that may be present are cystine, tyrosine, leucine, cholesterol, and sulfa. Crystals can be identified by their appearance and, if necessary, by their solubility characteristics (refer to Table 3-1). Since crystal formation tends to be pH-dependent, it is helpful to be aware of the pH of the urine when performing the microscopic examination.

Acid Urine

Those crystals which are frequently found in acid urine are uric acid, calcium oxalate, and amorphous urates (Fig. 3-11). Crystals which occur less frequently include: calcium sulfate, sodium urates, hippuric acid, cystine, leucine, tyrosine, cholesterol, and sulfa (Fig. 3-12).

URIC ACID CRYSTALS

Uric acid crystals can occur in many different shapes, but the most characteristic forms are the diamond or rhombic prism (Fig. 3-13), and the rosette (Fig. 3-14), which consists of many crystals clustered together. They may occasionally have six sides (Fig. 3-15) and this form is sometimes erroneously identified as cystine. (Cystine crystals are colorless.) Uric acid crystals are usually stained with urinary pigments and are, therefore, yellow or red-brown in color. The color is frequently dependent upon the thickness of the crystal, so very thin crystals may be colorless.

Under polarized light, uric acid crystals will take on a variety of colors. The polarized crystal in Figure 3-16 also demonstrates the layered effect that many uric acid crystals manifest. These crystals are soluble in sodium hydroxide, and insoluble in alcohol, hydrochloric acid, and acetic acid.

The presence of uric acid crystals in the urine can be a normal occurrence. It does not necessarily indicate a pathologic condition, nor does it mean that the uric acid content of the urine is definitely increased (Frankel 1963b). Pathologic conditions in which uric acid crystals are found in the urine include gout, high purine metabolism, acute febrile conditions, chronic nephritis, and Lesch-Nyhan syndrome (Sisson 1976).

(Continues on page 89)

TABLE 3-1

Properties of Crystalline Compounds

	pH		Solubility Properties
	Acid	**Alk**	
Amorphous urates	+	−	S—alkali, 60°C I—acetic acid
Bilirubin	+	−	S—chloroform, acid, alkali, acetone I—alcohol, ether
Calcium oxalates	+	±	S—HCl I—acetic acid
Calcium sulfate	+	−	S—acetic acid
Cholesterol	+	−	S—chloroform, ether, hot alcohol I—alcohol
Cystine	+	−	S—HCl, alkali, especially ammonia I—boiling H_2O, acetic acid, alcohol, ether
Hippuric acid	+	±	S—hot H_2O, alkali I—acetic acid
Leucine	+	−	S—hot acetic acid, hot alcohol, alkali I—HCl
Sodium urate	+	−	S—60°C sl. S—acetic acid
Sulfonamides	+	−	S—acetone
Tyrosine	+	−	S—NH_4OH, HCl, dilute mineral oil I—acetic acid, alcohol, ether
Uric acid	+	−	S—alkali I—alcohol, HCl, acetic acid
X-ray dye	+	−	S—10% NaOH
Ammonium biurates	±	+	S—60°C, acetic acid, strong alkali, NaOH (ammonia liberated)
Amorphous phosphates	−	+	S—acetic acid
Calcium carbonate	−	+	S—acetic acid (effervescence)
Calcium phosphates	−	+	S—dilute acetic acid
Triple phosphates	−	+	S—dilute acetic acid

± Crystals may be present at this pH, although they are more common at
  the other pH.
S = Soluble
I = Insoluble

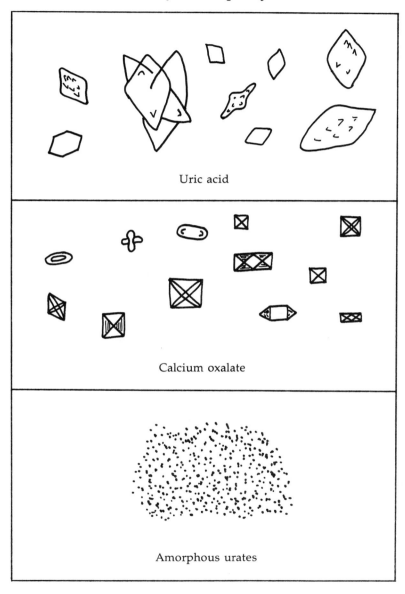

Uric acid

Calcium oxalate

Amorphous urates

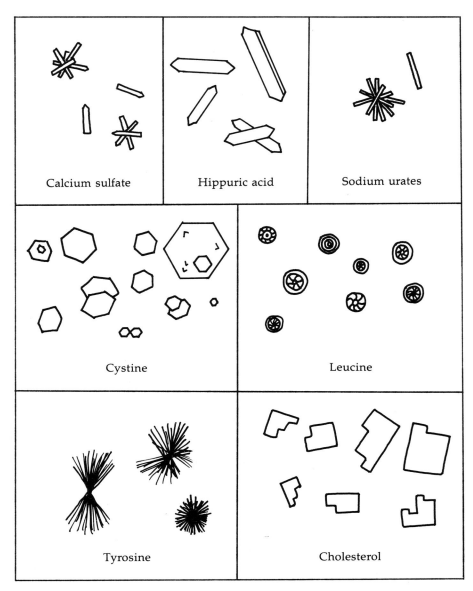

FIGURE 3-12   **Other crystals found in acid urine.**

FIGURE 3-13   **Uric acid crystals.**   Diamond or rhombic prism form. (500 ×). ▶

FIGURE 3-14   **Uric acid crystals in rosette formation.** (500 ×). ▶

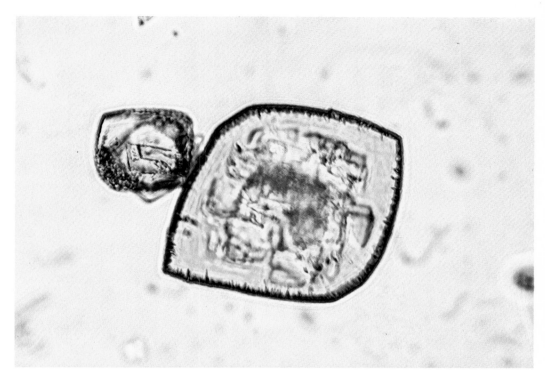

Fig. 3-13

Fig. 3-14

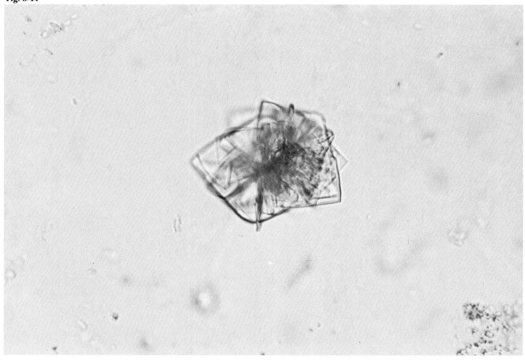

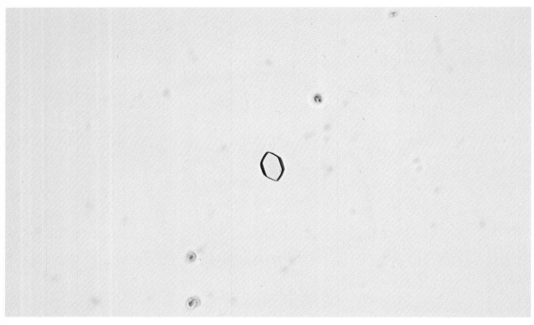

FIGURE 3-15   **Six-sided uric acid crystal.** (400×).

FIGURE 3-16   **Polarized uric acid crystal.**   Note the layered or laminated surface. (400×).

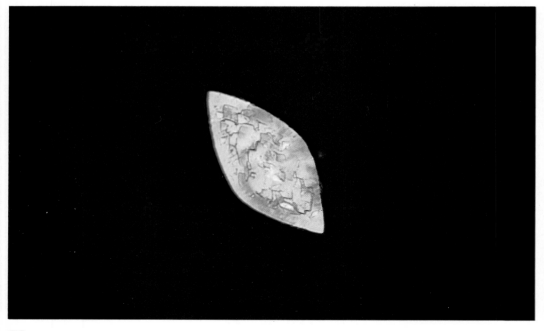

CALCIUM OXALATE CRYSTALS

Calcium oxalate crystals are colorless octahedral or "envelope" shaped crystals which look like small squares crossed by intersecting diagonal lines (Fig. 3-17). Rarely, they also appear as oval spheres or biconcave disks which have a dumbbell shape when viewed from the side. These crystals can vary in size, so that at times they are only barely discernible under high power magnification. When focusing on the typical calcium oxalate crystal, the viewer will see the "X" of the crystal popping out of the field (Fig. 3-18).

Calcium oxalate crystals are frequently found in acid and neutral urine, and occasionally they are also found in alkaline urine. They are soluble in hydrochloric acid but insoluble in acetic acid.

Calcium oxalate crystals can be present normally in the urine especially after the ingestion of various oxalate-rich foods such as tomatoes, spinach, rhubarb, garlic, oranges, and asparagus. Increased amounts of calcium oxalates, particularly if they are present in freshly voided urine, suggest the possibility of oxalate calculi. Other pathologic conditions in which calcium oxalates can be present in increased numbers include: ethylene glycol poisoning, diabetes mellitus, liver disease, and severe chronic renal disease.

Calcium oxalate crystals may be present in the urine following the intake of large doses of vitamin C. Oxalic acid is one of the breakdown products of ascorbic acid, and oxalic acid precipitates

Calcium oxalate crystals. (400 ×). **FIGURE 3-17**

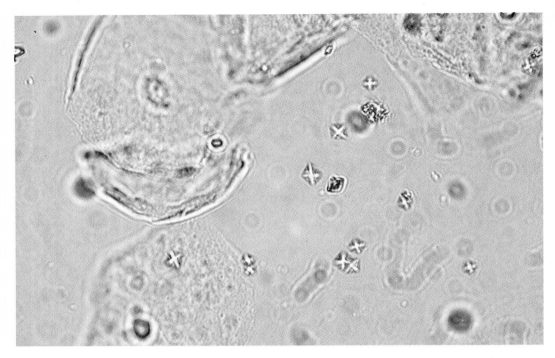

FIGURE 3-18   **Calcium oxalate crystals and squamous epithelial cells.**   The "X" of each crystal is very prominent. (500 ×).

ionized calcium (Krupp et al. 1979). This precipitation may also result in a decrease in the level of serum calcium.

AMORPHOUS URATES

Urate salts of sodium, potassium, magnesium, and calcium are frequently present in the urine in a noncrystalline, amorphous form. These amorphous urates have a yellow-red granular appearance (Fig. 3-19), and are soluble in alkali and at 60°C. They have no clinical significance.

HIPPURIC ACID CRYSTALS

These crystals are yellow-brown or colorless elongated prisms or plates (Fig. 3-20). They may be so thin as to resemble needles, and they often cluster together. Hippuric acid crystals are more soluble in water and ether than are uric acid crystals (Frankel 1963b). These crystals are rarely seen in the urine and have practically no clinical significance.

SODIUM URATES

Sodium urates may be present as amorphous or as crystals (Fig. 3-21). The sodium urate crystals are colorless or yellowish needles or slender prisms occurring in sheaves or clusters. They are soluble

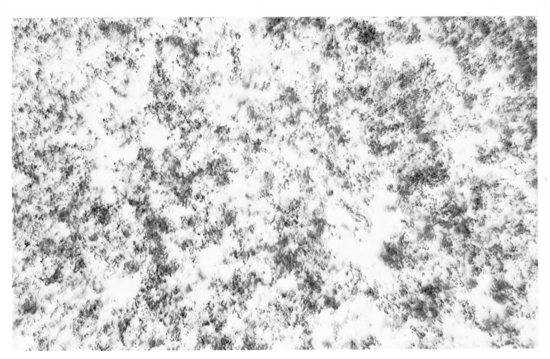

Amorphous urates. (200×). **FIGURE 3-19**

Hippuric acid crystal. (400×). **FIGURE 3-20**

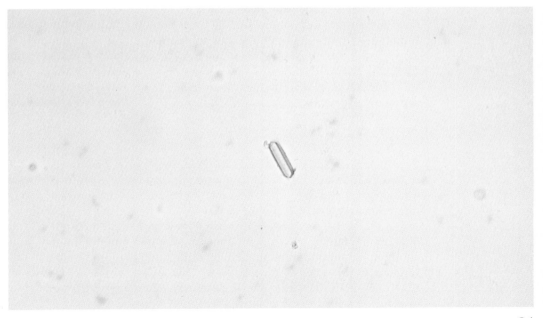

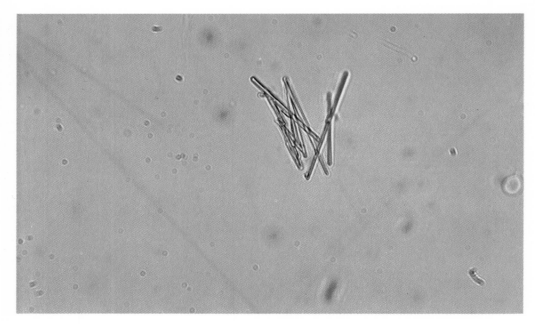

FIGURE 3-21 **Sodium urate crystals.** These needle-like crystals are not pointed at the ends. (400×).

at 60°C and only slightly soluble in acetic acid. Sodium urates have no clinical significance.

CALCIUM SULFATE CRYSTALS

Calcium sulfate crystals are long, thin, colorless needles or prisms which are identical in appearance to calcium phosphate. The pH of the urine helps to differentiate these two crystals, because calcium sulfate is found in acid urine, whereas calcium phosphate is usually found in alkaline urine. Calcium sulfate is also extremely soluble in acetic acid. Calcium sulfate crystals are rarely seen in the urine and they have no clinical significance.

CYSTINE CRYSTALS

Cystine crystals are colorless, refractile, hexagonal plates with equal or unequal sides (Fig. 3-22). They may appear singly, on top of each other, or in clusters. Cystine crystals frequently have a layered or laminated appearance (Fig. 3-23).

Cystine crystals are insoluble in acetic acid, alcohol, acetone, ether, and boiling water. They are soluble in hydrochloric acid and alkali, especially ammonia. The solubility in ammonia helps to differentiate cystine from colorless, six-sided uric acid crystals (ROCOM 1975). Cystine can be detected chemically with the sodium cyanide–sodium nitroprusside test (see Chapter 5).

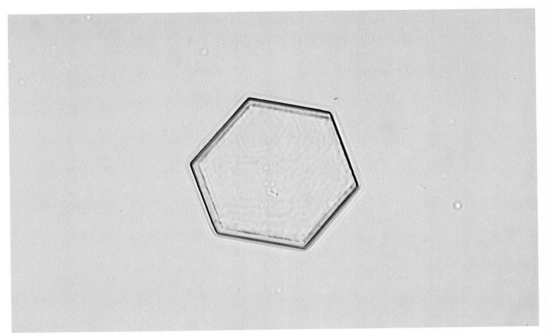

Cystine crystal. (1000 ×). **FIGURE 3-22**

Cystine crystals. Several have laminated surfaces. (160 ×). **FIGURE 3-23**

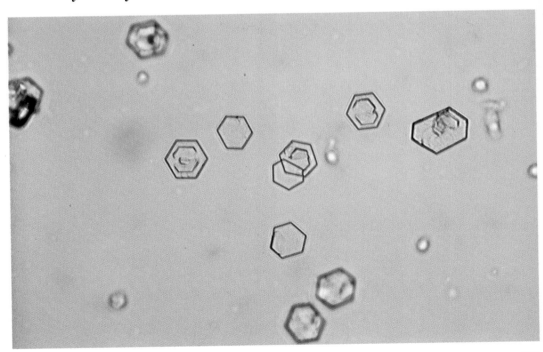

The presence of cystine crystals in the urine is always important. They occur in patients with either congenital cystinosis or congenital cystinuria, and they can form calculi.

LEUCINE
Leucine crystals are oily, highly refractile, yellow or brown spheroids with radial and concentric striations (Fig. 3-24). These spheroids are probably not pure leucine, because pure leucine crystallizes out as plates (Bradley et al. 1979). Leucine is soluble in hot acetic acid, hot alcohol, and in alkali, but insoluble in hydrochloric acid.

Leucine crystals are clinically very significant. They are found in the urine of patients with maple syrup urine disease, Oasthouse urine disease (Sisson 1976), and in serious liver disease such as terminal cirrhosis of the liver, severe viral hepatitis, and acute yellow atrophy of the liver. Leucine and tyrosine crystals are frequently present together in the urine of patients with liver disease.

TYROSINE
Tyrosine crystals are very fine, highly refractile needles occurring in sheaves or clusters (Figs. 3-25, and 3-26). The needle clusters often

FIGURE 3-24 **Leucine spheroids and WBCs.** Stained sediment. (Courtesy of Medcom, Inc., New York City.)

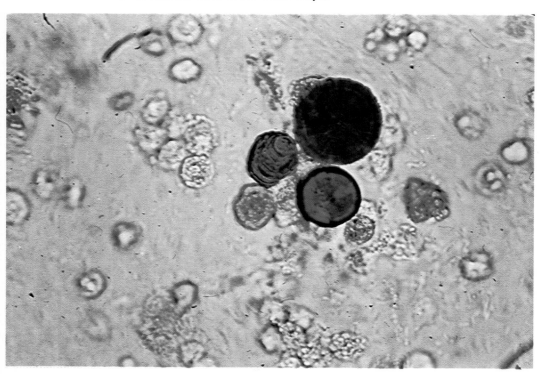

Tyrosine crystals. (160×). FIGURE 3-25

Same tyrosine crystals as Figure 3-25, but under a higher power. Note the fine, highly refractile needles that are typical of these crystals. (1000×). FIGURE 3-26

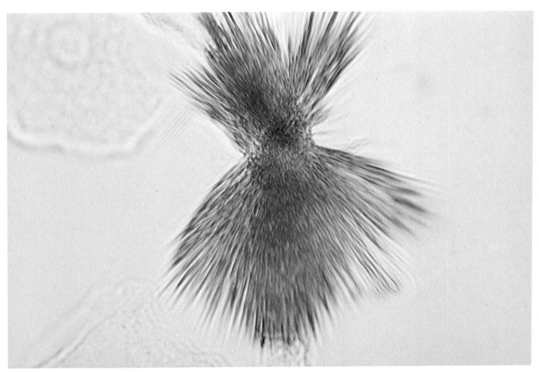

appear to be black, especially in the center, but they may take on a yellow color in the presence of bilirubin. Tyrosine crystals are soluble in ammonium hydroxide and hydrochloric acid, but insoluble in acetic acid.

Tyrosine crystals occur in severe liver disease, tyrosinosis, and Oasthouse urine disease.

CHOLESTEROL

Cholesterol crystals are large, flat, transparent plates with notched corners (Fig. 3-27). Under polarized light they may exhibit a variety of colors (Monte-Verde et al. 1979). They are soluble in chloroform, ether, and hot alcohol. At times, cholesterol crystals are found as a film on the surface of the urine instead of in the sediment (Frankel 1963b).

The presence of cholesterol plates (crystals) in the urine indicates excessive tissue breakdown (Krupp et al. 1979, Alba 1975), and these crystals are seen in nephritis and nephrotic conditions. They may also be present in chyluria (Frankel 1963b), which is the result of either thoracic or abdominal obstruction to lymph drainage, thereby

FIGURE 3-27   **Cholesterol crystal with typical notched edges.** (250×).

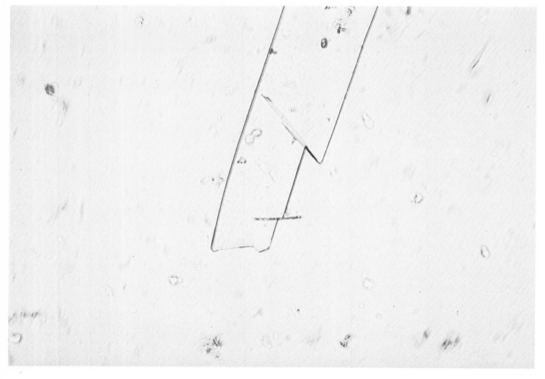

causing rupture of the lymphatic vessels into the renal pelvis or urinary tract. Some of the causes of obstruction to the lymphatic flow include tumors, gross enlargement of the abdominal lymph nodes, and filariasis.

SULFA AND OTHER DRUG CRYSTALS

When sulfonamide drugs were first introduced, there were many problems with renal damage resulting from the precipitation of the drug. The newer sulfa drugs are much more soluble, even in an acid environment, and so now they rarely form crystals in the urine.

Most of the sulfonamide drugs precipitate out as sheaves of needles, usually with eccentric binding, and they may be clear or brown in color (Fig. 3-28). Two steps should be followed to confirm the presence of sulfa crystals. First, if possible, contact the nursing station (if the urine is from an inpatient) to verify that the patient is taking sulfa medication. Second, perform the lignin test for sulfonamides which is discussed in Chapter 5. Sulfonamide crystals are soluble in acetone.

Sulfonamide crystals. Stained sediment. Note the eccentric binding. (Courtesy of Medcom, Inc., New York City.)   **FIGURE 3-28**

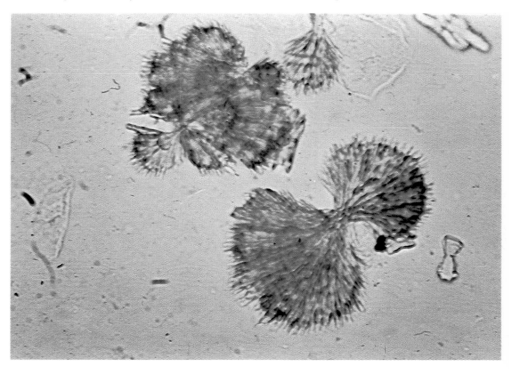

Radiographic dyes including Hypaque (Fig. 3-29) and Reno-grafin (Fig. 3-30) (both dyes are diatrizoate meglumine plus diatrizoate sodium) can crystallize out in an acid urine following intravenous injection for x-ray studies. Both of these dyes crystallize out as pleomorphic needles which can occur singly or in sheaves. The needles may be quite large, are often seen with brown spheres (Fig. 3-31), and will polarize light (Fig. 3-32). Radiographic dyes are very dense, and, when present in the urine, will result in an elevated specific gravity. The presence of needle crystals in a urine with a grossly elevated specific gravity (often >1.050) is usually indicative of x-ray dye. Radiographic dyes may be present in the urine for up to three days following injection.

The administration of large parenteral doses of ampicillin can result in the drug precipitating out as masses of long, thin, colorless needles in acid urine. Other drugs can occasionally result in the formation of crystals if administered in very large doses.

In some cases of bilirubinuria, the bilirubin may crystallize out in acid urine as red or reddish-brown needles or granules (Fig. 3-33). Bilirubin crystals are readily soluble in chloroform, acetone, acid, and alkali but are insoluble in alcohol and ether (ROCOM 1975). These crystals are of no more significance than the fact that bilirubin is present in the urine.

FIGURE 3-29   **X-ray dye crystals (Hypaque).** (160×).

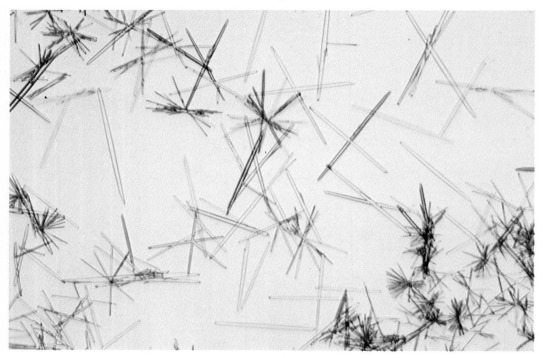

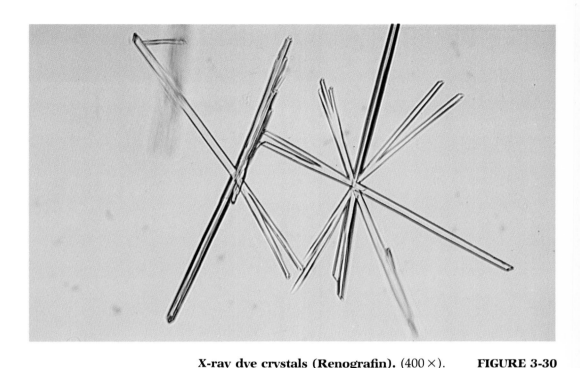

X-ray dye crystals (Renografin). $(400\times)$.　　　**FIGURE 3-30**

X-ray dye crystals (Hypaque).　Radiographic dyes are　　**FIGURE 3-31**
frequently accompanied by brown spheres. $(160\times)$.

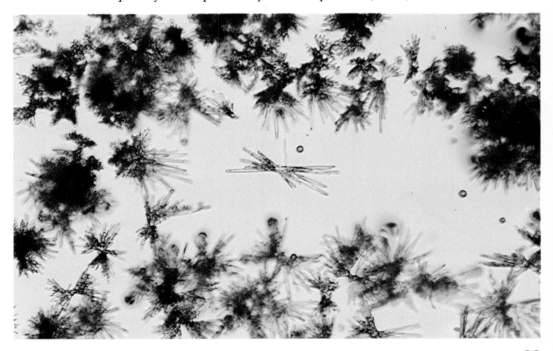

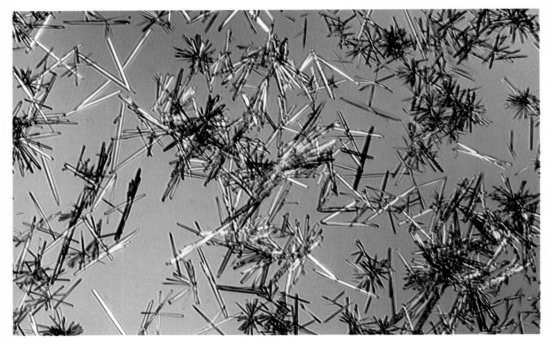

FIGURE 3-32   **Polarized x-ray dye crystals.** $(160 \times)$.

FIGURE 3-33   **Bilirubin crystals.** $(500 \times)$.

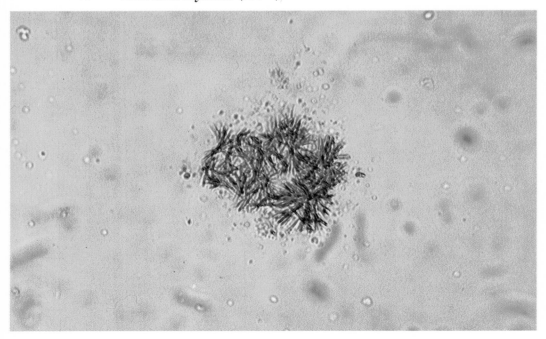

Alkaline Urine

Those crystals which can be found in alkaline urine include the following: triple phosphates (ammonium magnesium phosphates), amorphous phosphates, calcium carbonate, calcium phosphate, and ammonium biurates (also called ammonium urates) (Fig. 3-34).

Crystals found in alkaline urine.   **FIGURE 3-34**

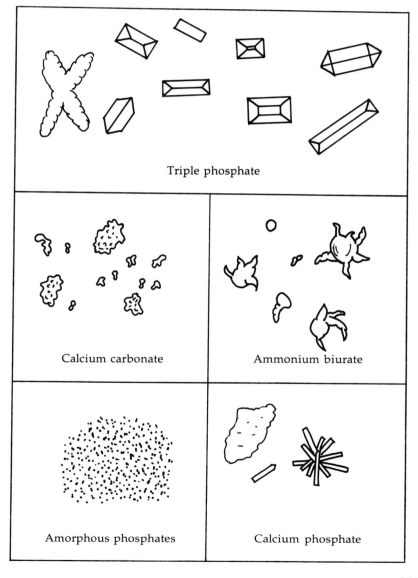

Triple phosphate

Calcium carbonate

Ammonium biurate

Amorphous phosphates

Calcium phosphate

TRIPLE PHOSPHATES

Triple phosphate (ammonium magnesium phosphate) crystals can be present in neutral and alkaline urines. The crystals are colorless prisms with from three to six sides which frequently have oblique ends (Fig. 3-35). Triple phosphates may sometimes precipitate in feathery or fern-like crystals. Triple phosphate crystals are soluble in acetic acid.

These crystals are frequently found in normal urine, but they can also form urinary calculi. Pathologic conditions in which they may be found include chronic pyelitis, chronic cystitis, enlarged prostate, and when the urine is retained in the bladder (Frankel 1963b).

AMORPHOUS PHOSPHATES

Phosphate salts are frequently present in the urine in a noncrystal-line, amorphous form (Fig. 3-36). These granular particles have no definite shape and they are usually visibly indistinguishable from amorphous urates. The pH of the urine helps to distinguish between

FIGURE 3-35   **Triple phosphate crystals.**   Note the oblique ends of the prisms. (200×).

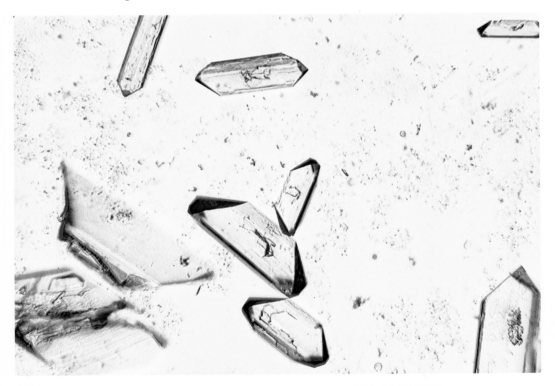

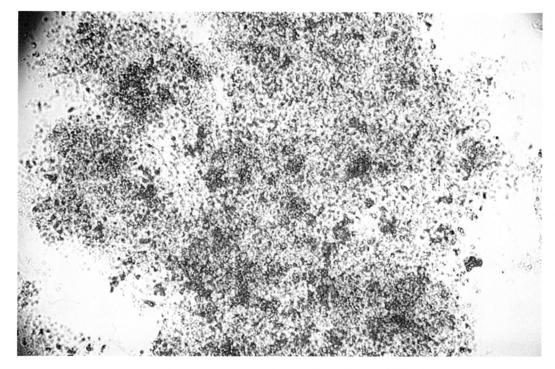

Amorphous phosphates. $(400 \times)$.   **FIGURE 3-36**

these two amorphous deposits as well as does their solubility properties. Amorphous phosphates are soluble in acetic acid, whereas amorphous urates are insoluble. Amorphous phosphates have no clinical significance.

CALCIUM CARBONATE

Calcium carbonate crystals are small, colorless crystals appearing in dumbbell or spherical forms, or in large granular masses (Fig. 3-37). They are larger than amorphous and, when in clumps, they may appear to have a dark color. The mass of calcium carbonate crystals, as opposed to a clump of amorphous phosphates, will also be connected together around the edges.

Calcium carbonate crystals have no clinical significance, and they will dissolve in acetic acid with the resulting evolution of carbon dioxide gas.

CALCIUM PHOSPHATE

Calcium phosphate crystals are long, thin, colorless prisms with one pointed end, arranged as rosettes or stars (stellar phosphates), or appearing as needles (Fig. 3-38). They may also form large, thin,

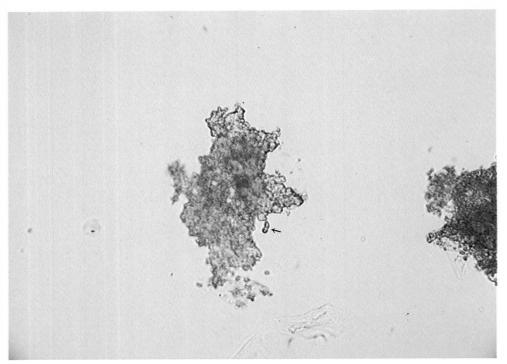

Fig. 3-37

Fig. 3-38

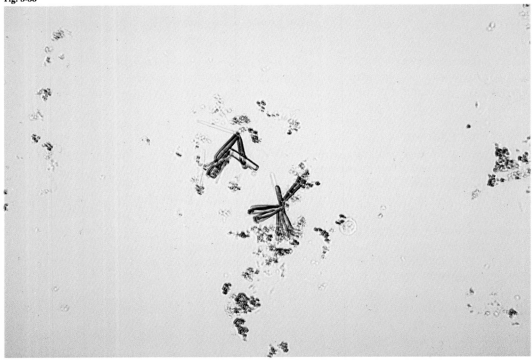

3. MICROSCOPIC EXAMINATION OF THE URINARY SEDIMENT

◄ **Calcium carbonate crystals (*center*).**   The *small arrow* points out the typical "dumbbell" form which is next to a large mass of calcium carbonate crystals. Note the difference between the calcium carbonate crystals and the clump of amorphous phosphates *on the right* of the picture. (400×).

FIGURE 3-37

◄ **Calcium phosphate crystals.** (400×).

FIGURE 3-38

---

irregular, granular plates which may float on the surface of the urine (Fig. 3-39). Calcium phosphates are soluble in dilute acetic acid. They may be present in normal urine, but they may also form calculi.

AMMONIUM BIURATES

Ammonium biurate crystals, which are also referred to as ammonium urates, are found in alkaline and neutral urine and occasionally they may be in acid urine (Frankel 1963b, ROCOM 1975). Ammonium biurates are yellow-brown spherical bodies with long, irregular spicules (Fig. 3-40). Their appearance is often described with the term "thorn apple". Ammonium biurates may also occur as yellow-

Calcium phosphate plate or phosphate sheath. (200×).

FIGURE 3-39

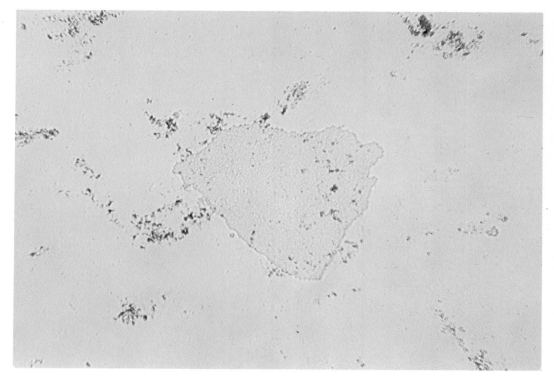

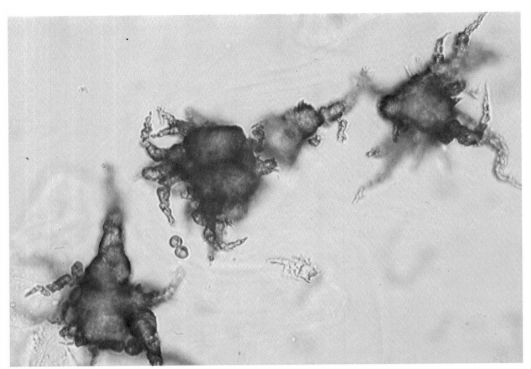

Fig. 3-40

Fig. 3-41

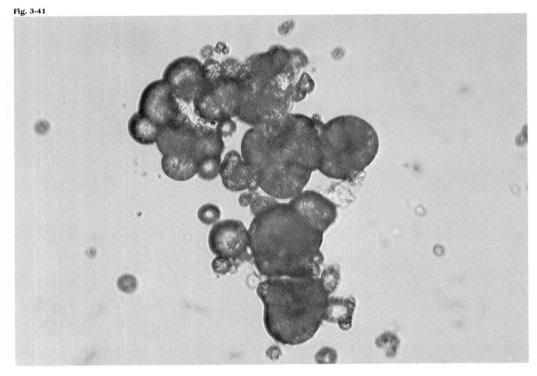

3. MICROSCOPIC EXAMINATION OF THE URINARY SEDIMENT

brown spheroids without spicules (Fig. 3-41), although this form is not that common.

Ammonium biurates dissolve by warming and are soluble in acetic acid, with the formation of colorless uric acid crystals after standing. The addition of sodium hydroxide will liberate ammonia (Bauer et al. 1968). Ammonium biurates are only abnormal if found in freshly voided urine (Hepler 1949).

Casts

Urinary casts are formed in the lumen of the tubules of the kidney. They are so named because they are molded in the tubules. Casts can form as the result of the precipitation or gelation of Tamm-Horsfall mucoprotein (McQueen 1966, Rutecki et al. 1971), the clumping of cells or other material within a protein matrix (Haber 1976, Greenhill and Gruskin 1976), the adherence of cells or material to the matrix (Haber and Lindner 1977), or by conglutination of material within the lumen (Lippman 1957). The renal tubules secrete a mucoprotein called Tamm-Horsfall protein which is believed to form the basic matrix of all casts (McQueen 1966). Some casts may also contain serum proteins but they are usually confined to the cast granules (Rutecki et al. 1971). In waxy casts, serum proteins are present in a homogeneous distribution (Schreiner 1969).

Factors that are involved in cast formation include urinary stasis (marked decrease in urine flow), increased acidity, high solute concentration, and the presence of abnormal ionic or protein constituents. Cast formation usually takes place in the distal and collecting tubules because there the urine reaches its maximum concentration and acidification (Weller 1979, Ravel 1978, Sweeney and Forland 1980). Casts will dissolve in alkaline urine (Burton and Rowe 1975) and in neutral urine having a specific gravity of 1.003 or less (Schreiner 1957). The presence of casts in the urine is frequently accompanied by proteinuria, but casts can be seen in the absence of protein (Bauer et al. 1968).

Casts have nearly parallel sides and rounded or blunted ends, and they vary in size and shape according to the tubules in which they were formed. They may be convoluted, straight, or curved, and they may vary in length. The width of the cast indicates the diameter of the tubule responsible for its formation. Broad casts, which can be from two to six times wider than ordinary casts (Hoffman 1970, Sisson 1976), are formed either in pathologically dilated or atrophied tubules, or in collecting tubules. Broad casts are frequently referred to as renal failure casts.

Casts are always renal in origin, and they are important indicators of intrinsic renal disease. They may be present in glomerular damage, tubular damage, renal inflammation, and renal infection. Casts are classified on the basis of their appearance and the cellular components which they may contain. The different types of casts are: hyaline, red cell, white cell, epithelial cell, granular (coarse and fine), waxy, and fatty. At times, it may be difficult to distinguish the various casts because of degeneration, or because the cast may contain a variety of structures (mixed casts). It has been proposed that as cellular casts degenerate they form granular casts that in turn degenerate, forming waxy casts. However, there seem to be several problems with this hypothesis (Rutecki et al. 1971, Haber and Lindner 1977).

Casts are cylindrical in shape and do not have dark edges. Occasionally, waxy casts may appear to have a thin dark edge but only because the shiny surface of the cast comes to an abrupt ending. Usually this thin dark edge will disappear when the fine adjustment is turned slightly. Any structure, therefore, that has dark edges is most likely a piece of fiber. Also, any structure with parallel sides that is flat in the middle with thick edges is probably also a fiber. Remember, tubules are round, so casts will be more or less circular, and will be thicker in the middle.

Casts are reported according to type and the number that is present per low power field (100×).

Hyaline Casts

Hyaline casts are the most frequently occurring casts in the urine. They are composed of gelled Tamm-Horsfall protein and may contain some inclusions which were incorporated while in the kidney. Since they are composed of only protein, they have a very low refractive index and must be viewed under low light. They are colorless, homogeneous, and transparent, and usually have rounded ends (Fig. 3-42).

Hyaline casts can be seen in even the mildest kind of renal disease, and are not associated with any one disease in particular (Haber 1976). A few hyaline casts may be found in the normal urine, and increased amounts are frequently present following physical exercise (Bailey et al. 1976), Haber et al. 1979) and physiologic dehydration (Cannon 1979).

Red Cell Casts

Red cell casts mean renal hematuria and they are always pathologic. They are usually diagnostic of glomerular disease being found in acute glomerulonephritis, lupus nephritis, Goodpasture's syndrome, subacute bacterial endocarditis, and renal trauma. Red cell casts can also be present in renal infarction, severe pyelonephritis, right-sided

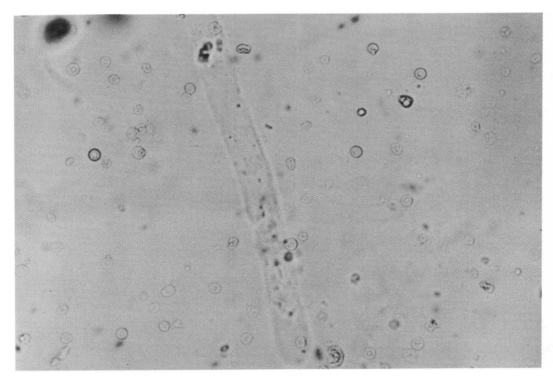

Hyaline cast and red blood cells. Note the low refractive index of the cast. (400×).

FIGURE 3-42

congestive heart failure, renal vein thrombosis, and periarteritis nodosa.

Red cell casts may appear brown to almost colorless (Fig. 3-43). The cast may contain only a few RBCs in a protein matrix, or there may be many cells packed close together with no visible matrix. If the red cells are still intact and the outlines are still detectable, then the cast is termed a red cell cast. If the cast has degenerated to a reddish-brown granular cast, then the cast is a hemoglobin or blood cast.

White Cell Casts

White cell casts are present in renal infection and in noninfectious inflammation. They can, therefore, be seen in acute pyelonephritis, interstitial nephritis, and lupus nephritis. They may also be present in glomerular disease.

The majority of white cells that appear in casts are polymorphonuclear neutrophils. The WBCs in the cast may be few in number, or there may be many cells tightly packed together (Fig. 3-44). If the cells are still intact, the nuclei may be clearly visible, but as they

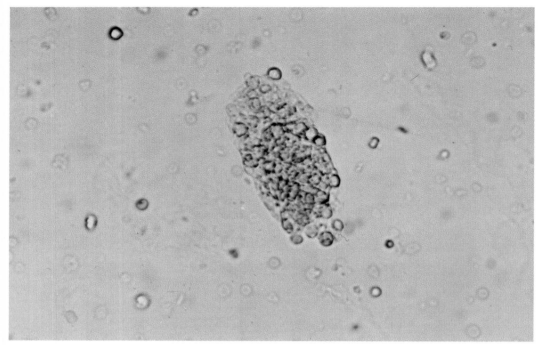

Fig. 3-43

Fig. 3-44

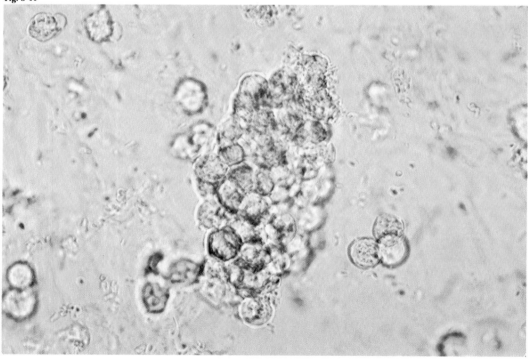

begin to degenerate, the cell membranes disappear and the cast becomes granular in appearance.

Granular Casts

Granular casts may be either the result of the degeneration of cellular casts, or they may represent the direct aggregation of serum proteins into a matrix of Tamm-Horsfall mucoprotein (Rutecki et al. 1971). Initially, the granules are large and coarse, but when urine stasis is prolonged, these granules break down to fine granules. Granular casts almost always indicate significant renal disease (Bradley et al. 1979), however, granular casts may be present in the urine for a short time following strenuous exercise (Rutecki et al. 1971).

Determining whether a cast is coarsely or finely granular is of no clinical significance, although the distinction is not hard to make (Haber 1976). Finely granular casts contain fine granules which may appear gray or pale yellow in color (Fig. 3-45). Coarsely granular casts contain larger granules that are darker in color and these casts often appear black because of the density of the granules (Fig. 3-46).

Epithelial Cell Casts

Epithelial cell casts form as the result of stasis and the desquamation of renal tubular epithelial cells. These casts are only rarely seen in the urine because of the infrequent occurrence of renal diseases which primarily affect the tubules (necrosis) (Haber 1976). Epithelial cell casts may be present in the urine after exposure to nephrotoxic agents or viruses (e.g., cytomegalovirus, hepatitis virus) which cause tubular degeneration and necrosis. These casts can also occur in severe chronic renal disease in which tubular damage accompanies glomerular injury, and in the rejection of a kidney allograft.

The epithelial cells may either be arranged in parallel rows in the cast, or they may be arranged haphazardly, and vary in size, shape, and stage of degeneration (Fig. 3-47). The cells in the former type of arrangement are believed to come from the same segment of the tubule, whereas the irregular arrangement seems to indicate that the cells came from different portions of the tubule (Haber 1976, Bradley et al. 1979).

Waxy Casts

Waxy casts have a very high refractive index, are yellow, gray, or colorless, and have a smooth homogeneous appearance (Figs. 3-48, 3-49). They frequently occur as short broad casts with blunt or broken ends, and they often have cracked or serrated edges.

(Continues on page 115)

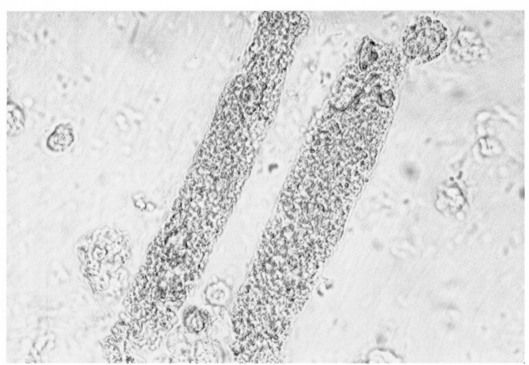

Fig. 3-45

Fig. 3-46

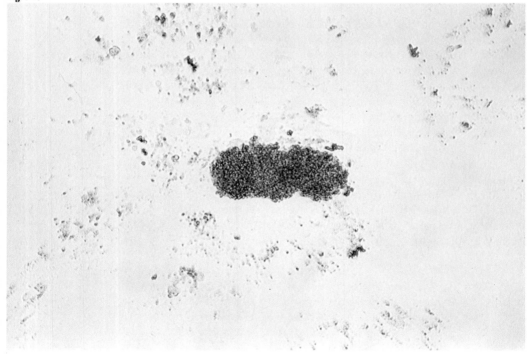

◄ **Finely granular casts.** Note the RBC between the two casts. (500×).   **FIGURE 3-45**

◄ **Broad coarsely granular cast.** (200×).   **FIGURE 3-46**

Epithelial cell cast. Field also contains triple phosphates and mucous threads. (200×).   **FIGURE 3-47**

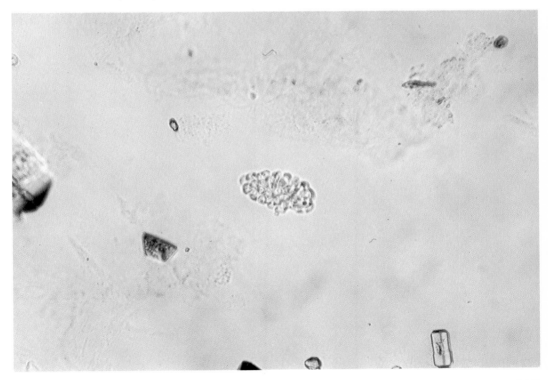

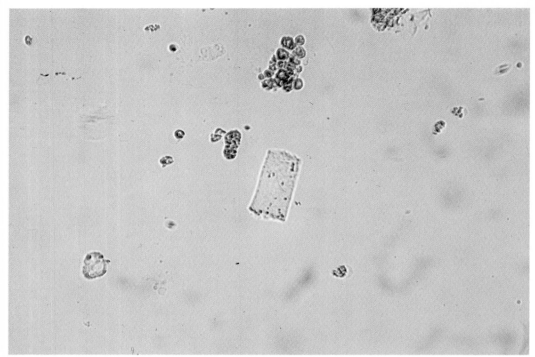
Fig. 3-48

Fig. 3-49
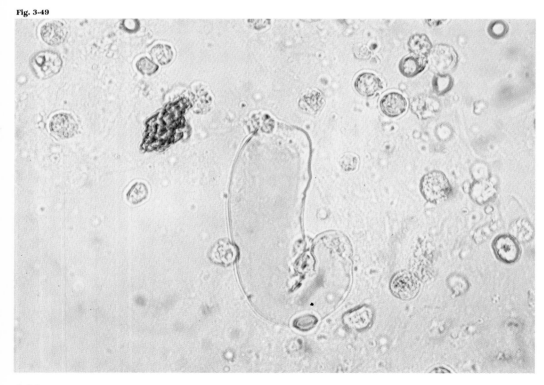

It has been postulated that waxy casts result from the degeneration of granular casts. Waxy casts are found in patients with severe chronic renal failure, malignant hypertension, renal amyloidosis, and diabetic nephropathy. They may also be found in acute renal disease, tubular inflammation and degeneration, and during renal allograft rejection.

Fatty Casts

Fatty casts are casts which have incorporated either free fat droplets or oval fat bodies (refer to the section on Oval Fat Bodies). These casts may contain only a few fat droplets, or the cast may be composed almost entirely of fat droplets of various sizes. Figure 3-50 shows a typical fatty cast with large fat droplets in half of the cast, and smaller yellow-brown droplets in the other half. If the fat is cholesterol, the droplets will be anisotropic, and under polarized light will demonstrate a characteristic "Maltese-cross" formation. Iso-

Fatty cast. (400 ×).   **FIGURE 3-50**

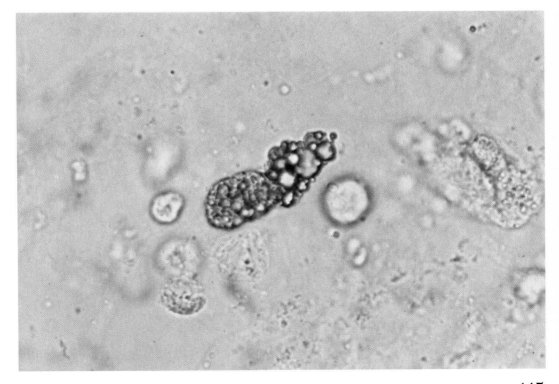

tropic droplets, which consist of triglycerides, will not polarize but will stain with Sudan III or Oil Red O.

Fatty casts are seen when there is fatty degeneration of the tubular epithelium, as in degenerative tubular disease. They are frequently seen in the nephrotic syndrome and may occur in diabetic glomerulosclerosis, lipoid nephrosis, chronic glomerulonephritis, Kimmelstiel-Wilson syndrome, lupus, and toxic renal poisoning.

Miscellaneous Structures

Other structures which may be present in the urine include bacteria, yeast, cylindroids, spermatozoa, mucous, and fat.

Bacteria

The urine is normally free of bacteria while in the kidney and bladder, but contamination may occur from bacteria present in the urethra or vagina, or from other external sources. When a properly collected, freshly voided specimen contains large numbers of bacteria, especially when accompanied by many white cells, it is usually indicative of a urinary tract infection. Bacteria are reported according to the

FIGURE 3-51   **Bacteria (rods, cocci, and chains).** (500×).

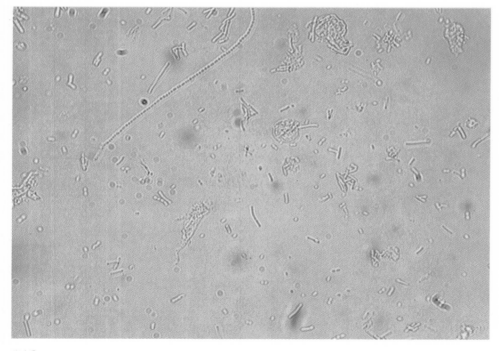

number that is present (few, moderate, etc.), but no attempt is made, in the routine urinalysis laboratory, to identify the exact organism.

The presence of bacteria is easily recognized when the sediment is viewed under high power magnification (Fig. 3-51).

Yeast

Yeast cells are smooth, colorless, usually ovoid cells with doubly refractile walls. They can vary in size and often show budding (Fig. 3-52). They may sometimes be mistaken for red cells, but unlike red cells, they are insoluble in acid and alkali, and they will not stain with eosin.

Yeast may be found in urinary tract infections, especially in diabetic patients. They may also be present in the urine as a result of skin or vaginal contamination. *Candida albicans* is the most common yeast to appear in the urine (Race and White 1979).

Cylindroids

Cylindroids resemble casts but have one end which tapers out like a strand of mucous. The exact site and mechanism of their formation

Yeast cells.   Note the budding and doubly refractile walls. (1000 ×).   FIGURE 3-52

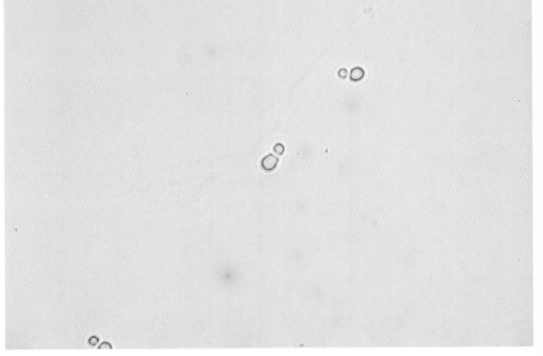

are not known, but since they usually occur in conjunction with casts, they are considered to have the same significance (Hepler 1949, Lippman 1957). Schreiner (1957) states that there is no longer a need for the separate classification of cylindroids from that of casts. Cylindroids are frequently hyaline, but like the one pictured in Figure 3-53, they may also incorporate other material.

Spermatozoa

Spermatozoa may be present in the urine of men after epileptic convulsions, nocturnal emissions, diseases of the genital organ, and in spermatorrhea. They may also be found in the urine of both sexes after coitus. Spermatozoa have oval bodies and long, thin, delicate tails (Fig. 3-54).

Mucous Threads

Mucous threads are long, thin, wavy threads of ribbon-like structures which may show faint longitudinal striations (Fig. 3-55). Mucous threads are present in normal urine in small numbers, but they may be very abundant in the presence of inflammation or irritation of the urinary tract. Some of the wider threads may be confused with

FIGURE 3-53   **Cylindroid.**   Note the tapering tail. (400 ×).

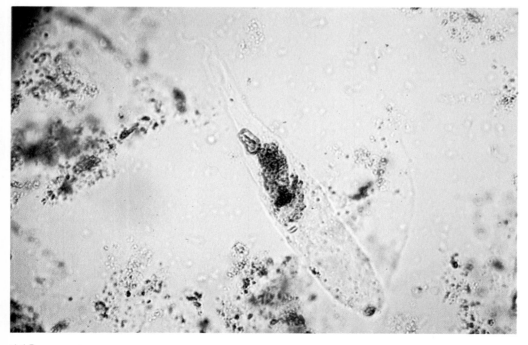

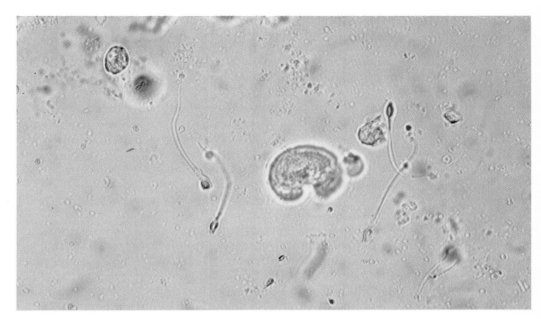

Spermatozoa. (500 ×). **FIGURE 3-54**

Mucous threads. Viewed with an 80A filter. (100 ×). **FIGURE 3-55**

cylindroids or hyaline casts. Heavy mucous threads tend to incorporate white cells.

Oval Fat Bodies and Free Fat Droplets

Fat may be present in the urine as free droplets or globules, within degenerating or necrotic cells (oval fat bodies), or incorporated in a cast.

Oval fat bodies are usually defined as being renal tubular cells which contain highly refractile fat droplets (Fig. 3-56). They are either the result of the incorporation of fat that has been filtered through the glomerulus, or they are renal tubular cells which have undergone fatty degeneration. Oval fat bodies may also be macrophages or polymorphonuclear leukocytes (Weller 1979, Latner 1975) which have either ingested lipids or degenerated cells, or have undergone fatty degeneration.

Lipids may also appear in the urine as free fat droplets (Fig. 3-57). These droplets frequently vary in size, since the fat globules can coalesce together. Fat droplets are highly refractile, are globular in shape, and frequently have a yellow-brown appearance, although under low power and under subdued light they may sometimes appear to be black because of their high refractive index. In lipuria (the excretion of lipids in the urine), the free fat droplets may be found floating on the surface of the urine.

If the fat droplets, whether floating free or incorporated in a cell or cast, are composed of cholesterol esters or free cholesterol, they will be anisotropic (Zimmer et al. 1961) and will form "Maltese crosses" under polarized light (Fig. 3-58), but they will not stain with fat stain. If they consist of triglycerides, or neutral fat, they will not polarize but will stain with Sudan III or Oil Red O (Bradley et al. 1979).

Anisotropic fat globules which manifest the "Maltese-cross" formation are termed "doubly refractile fat bodies" (Schreiner 1963).

Fat may be present in the urine as the result of fatty degeneration of the tubules. It is frequently found in the nephrotic syndrome, and may also be present in diabetes mellitus, eclampsia, toxic renal poisoning, chronic glomerulonephritis, lipoid nephrosis, fat embolism (Hansen et al. 1973), and following extensive superficial injuries with crushing of the subcutaneous fat (Latner 1975). Lipuria may also occur following fractures of the major long bones or pelvis, and in multiple fractures in which fat may be released from the bone marrow into the circulation and then filtered through the glomerulus.

FIGURE 3-56   **Oval fat body and a fiber.** (500×). ▶

FIGURE 3-57   **Fat droplets.**   Field also contains WBCs. (500×). ▶

120   **3. MICROSCOPIC EXAMINATION OF THE URINARY SEDIMENT**

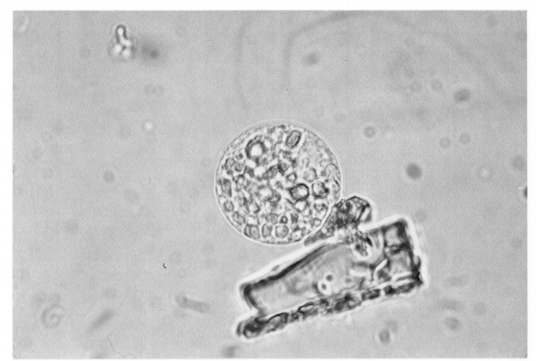

Fig. 3-56

Fig. 3-57

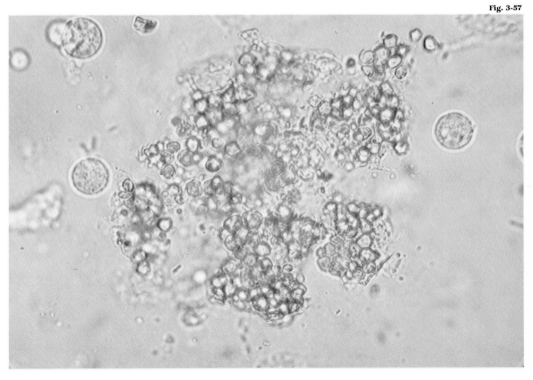

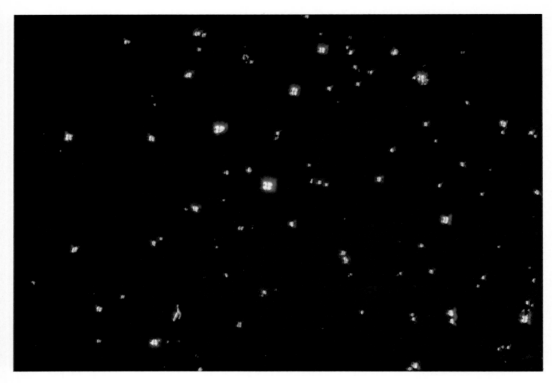

FIGURE 3-58 **Polarized anisotropic fat droplets.** Note the "Maltese-cross" formation. (160 ×).

Artifacts

A variety of foreign objects can find their way into the urine specimen during collection, transportation, while being tested, or while on the microscope slide. It is important that the technologist be able to recognize these objects as being extraneous structures.

Starch Crystals

Starch crystals are frequently found in the urine. They are round or oval, are highly refractive, and vary in size. The most common type of starch which can be present in the urine is cornstarch, possibly because some brands of powder contain cornstarch. Cornstarch crystals are almost hexagonal in shape, and they contain an irregular indentation in the center (Fig. 3-59). Under polarized light these starch crystals will appear as "Maltese crosses" (Fig. 3-60). Anisotropic fat and starch are the only structures that will form these crosses under polarized light.

Lycopodium is similar in appearance to cornstarch and is used as a dusting powder.

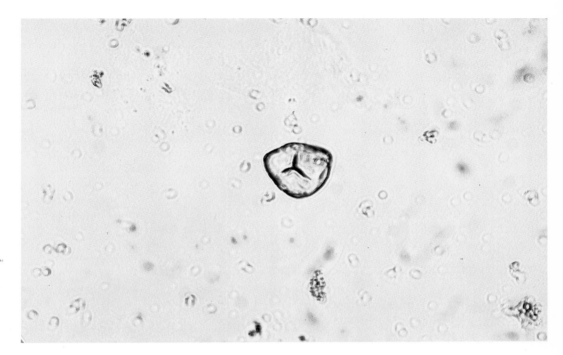

Starch crystal. (500 ×).   **FIGURE 3-59**

Polarized starch crystals.   Note the "Maltese-cross"   **FIGURE 3-60**
formation. (400 ×).

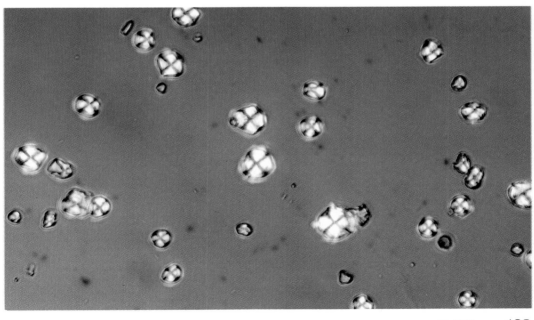

Fibers

Cloth fibers are undoubtedly the most frequently occurring type of artifact found in the urine. They may come from clothing, diapers, toilet paper, lens paper, or they may be pieces of lint from the air. Fibers which are long and flat are easily recognizable (Fig. 3-61). However, fibers which are short and are approximately the same size as casts are often mistaken for casts, even by some "urinalysis experts".

The author feels that this error can be avoided by exposing the technologist to the various types of fibers, because there are certain characteristics of the different fibers that can be easily recognized. The author recommends that the student or reader take a disposable diaper, cut a small square out of it, wet the section with water, squeeze it out into a test tube, and examine the sediment (Fig. 3-62). This is the same type of sediment that is obtained when the nursing personnel squeeze the urine out of a diaper. The disposable diaper contains many of the varieties of fibers which appear as contaminants in the urine specimen.

When observing the different fibers, a few characteristics can be readily noticeable. First of all, they usually have dark edges; casts do not have dark edges. Secondly, most of the fibers are flat; casts are

FIGURE 3-61   **Cloth fibers.** (160 ×).

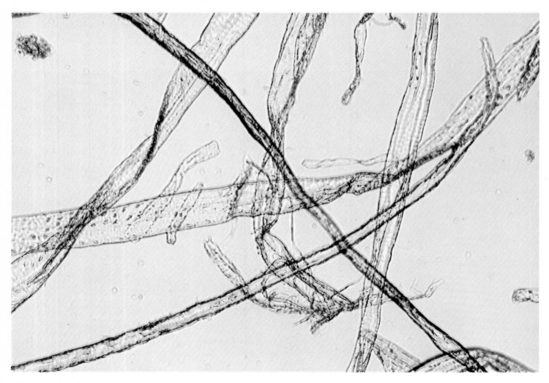

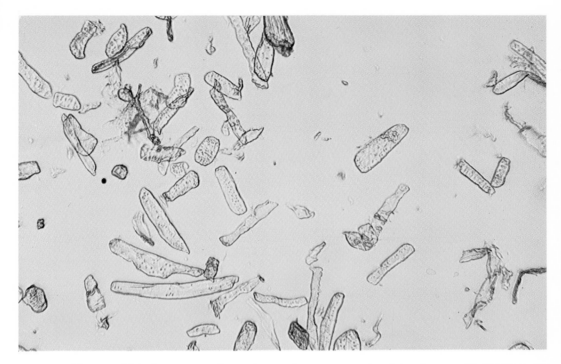

Fibers. This is an actual specimen that was received in the lab for microscopic examination. (200×).   **FIGURE 3-62**

cylindrical. The fiber in Figure 3-63 is frequently encountered in the urine sediment, but may be recognized by the thick, nodular edges and the nodular indentations on both ends of the fiber. This fiber is thicker on the edges than in the middle (clue), and is usually flat (another clue). Refer to the Atlas in Chapter 4 for more pictures of the various fibers.

Oil Droplets

Oil droplets in the urine are the result of contamination from lubricants. They are spherical and can vary in size (Fig. 3-64).

Miscellaneous Structures

Some of the other types of debris or extraneous material which may be found in the urinary sediment include: hair (Fig. 3-65); glass fragments (Fig. 3-66), as well as scratches on the microscope slide; air bubbles (Fig. 3-67); pollen granules; and talcum powder, which is usually formed from silicate sources and, thus, the particles have rather angular shapes (Fig. 3-68).

The urine may be contaminated with fecal material and may, therefore, contain vegetable fibers, muscle fibers, and tissue strands (Fig. 3-69). These structures should be recognized as being fecal contaminants. *(Continues on page 129)*

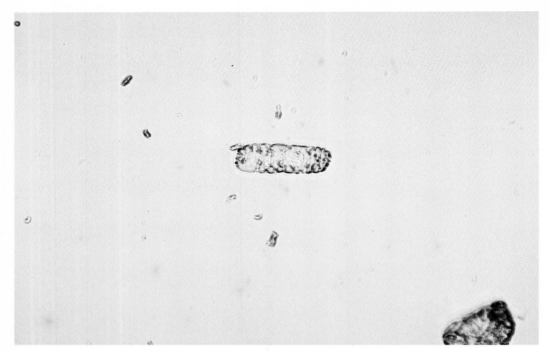

FIGURE 3-63   **Fiber.**   This fiber is a common contaminant. (400×).

FIGURE 3-64   **Oil droplet.**   Field also contains WBCs and squamous epithelial cells. (400×).

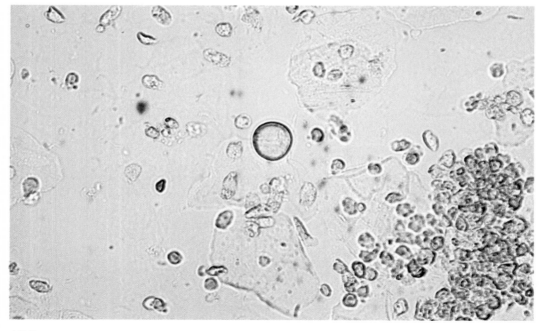

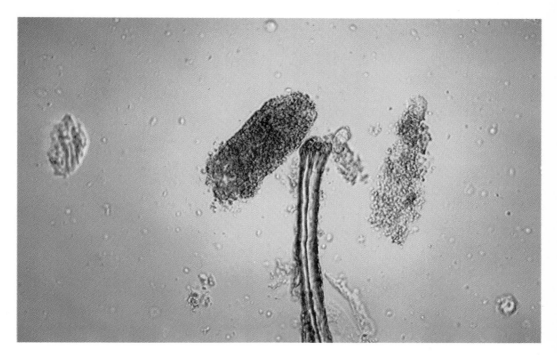

Hair and a coarsely granular cast. Viewed with an 80A   **FIGURE 3-65**
filter. (400×).

Glass fragments. These are frequently present if a glass   **FIGURE 3-66**
pipette is used to transfer the sediment to the slide. (400×).

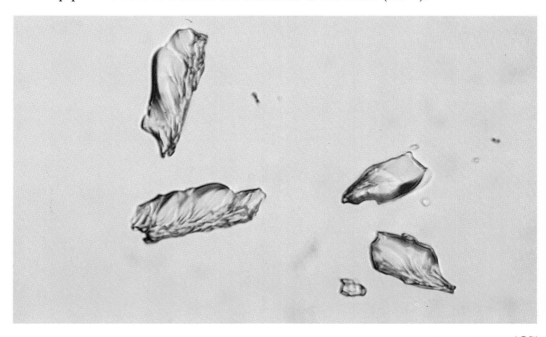

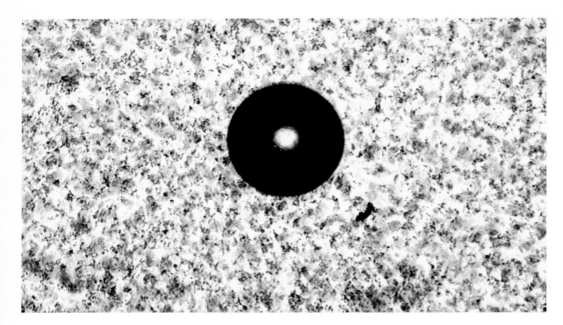

FIGURE 3-67   **Air bubble and amorphous urates.** $(160\times)$.

FIGURE 3-68   **Talcum powder particles.** $(160\times)$.

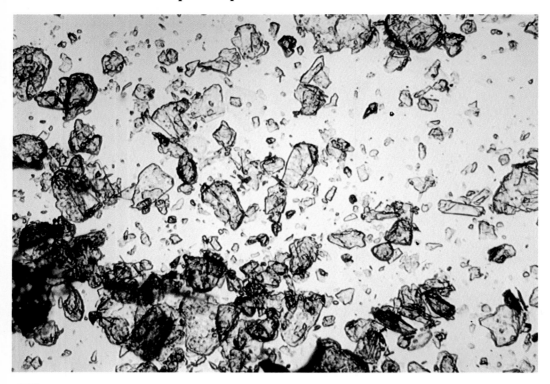

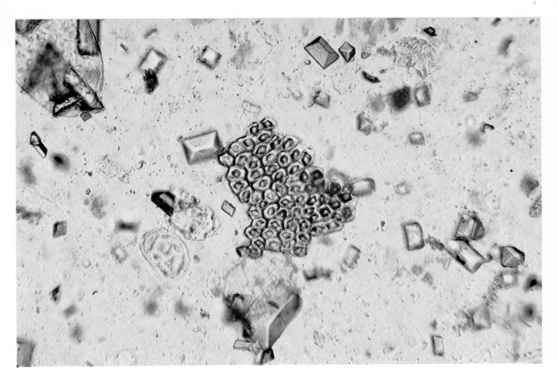

Fecal contamination. Field also contains triple phosphate crystals. (100×).   **FIGURE 3-69**

Parasites

Parasites may occasionally be found in the urine, either because they are indigenous to the urinary tract, or as the result of vaginal or fecal contamination.

Trichomonas vaginalis is the most frequently occurring parasite in the urine. It is a flagellate organism which is about the same size as a large white cell (Fig. 3-70). In the unstained wet mount, the organism should not be reported unless it is motile. Sometimes when bacteria are next to a white cell, the cell may be mistaken for *Trichomonas*, which is why motility is the diagnostic feature. This organism may be found in males, although it is more common in females. *Trichomonas vaginalis* is frequently accompanied by WBCs and epithelial cells.

Enterobius vermicularis (pinworm) ova and occasionally also the female adult may be found in the urine, perhaps even more frequently than was once believed. The ova are very characteristic in shape, having one flat and one rounded side (Fig. 3-71). The developing larva can usually be observed through the transparent shell of the egg. If the urine is found to contain many ova, examination of the original urine container may reveal the adult worm (Fig. 3-72).

(Continues on page 132)

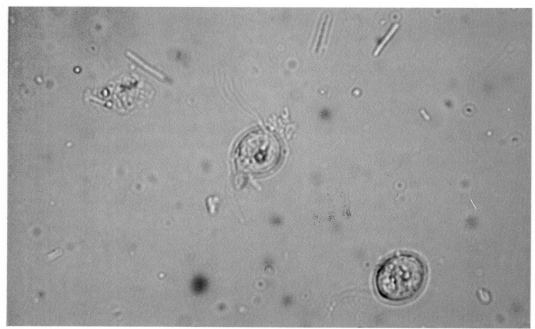

Fig. 3-70

Fig. 3-71

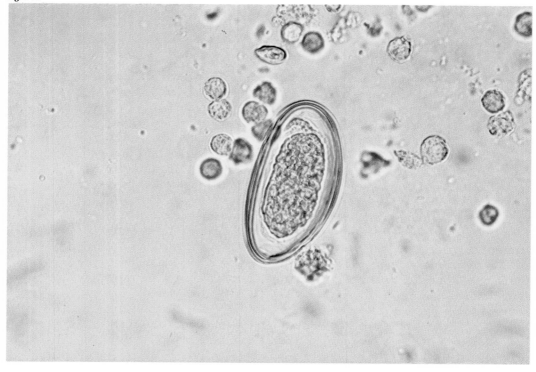

3. MICROSCOPIC EXAMINATION OF THE URINARY SEDIMENT

◀ *Trichomonas vaginalis.* Note the four flagella. (1000×).   **FIGURE 3-70**

◀ *Enterobius vermicularis* **ovum and WBCs.** (500×).   **FIGURE 3-71**

Head of the *Enterobius vermicularis* adult female worm.   **FIGURE 3-72**
(100×).

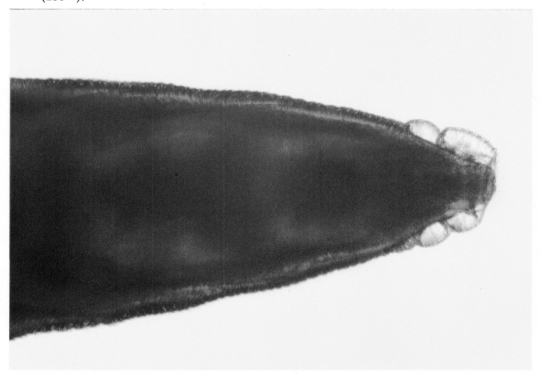

Schistosoma haematobium is a blood fluke that inhabits the veins in the wall of the urinary bladder. The adult deposits eggs in the capillaries of the mucosa. Abscesses develop around the eggs, and the eggs can be found in the urine accompanied by RBCs and WBCs. This type of schistosomiasis is endemic in Africa, especially around the Nile Valley, in the Middle East, and around the Mediterranean. The *Schistosoma haematobium* ovum has a characteristic terminal spine and measures about 50μ by 150μ (Fig. 3-73).

FIGURE 3-73   *Schistosoma haematobium* **ovum.**
(Courtesy of Dr. Kenneth A. Borchardt.)

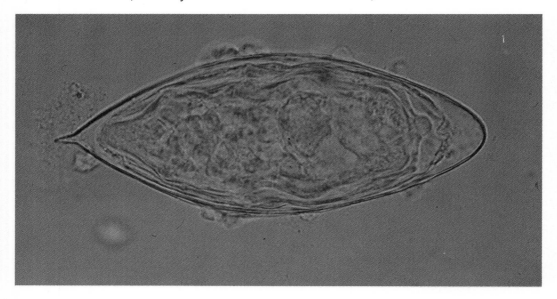

4

An Atlas of Urinary Sediment

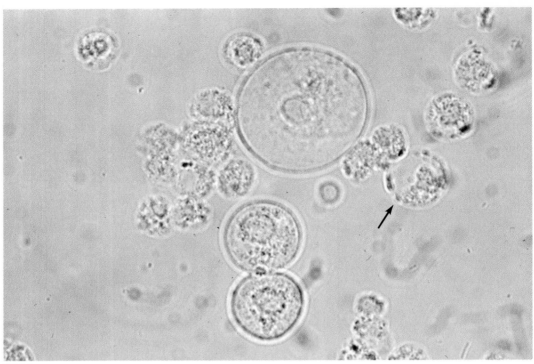

Fig. 4-1

Fig. 4-2

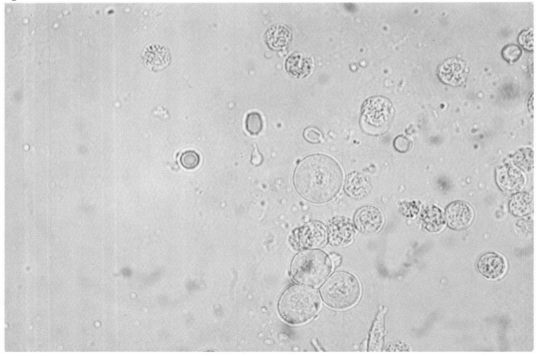

◀ **Hypotonic urine containing WBCs, 1 RBC, 2 renal epithelial cells, and a transitional epithelial cell.** Note the size of the swollen WBCs. The *arrow* indicates a WBC that is ready to lyse. (500×).

FIGURE 4-1

◀ **Epithelial cells, WBCs, RBCs, and bacteria.** The four epithelial cells may all be renal tubular cells, but the nuclei are indistinguishable on this focal plane. (500×).

FIGURE 4-2

Many RBCs and a squamous epithelial cell. (160×).

FIGURE 4-3

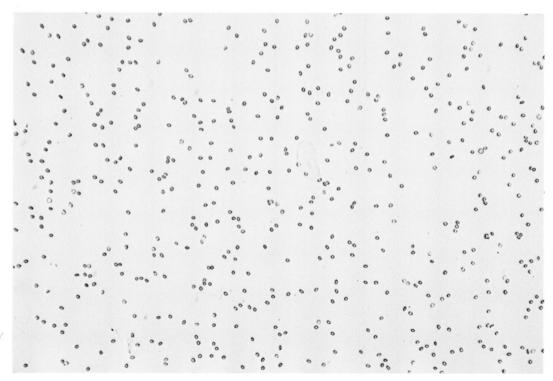

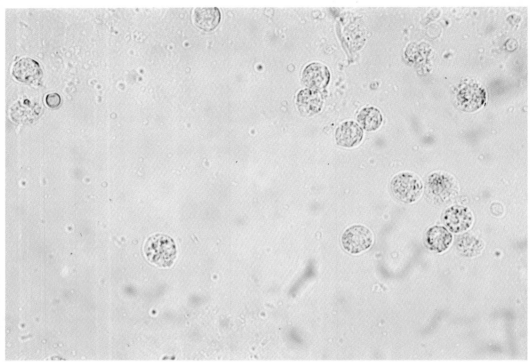

Fig. 4-4

Fig. 4-5

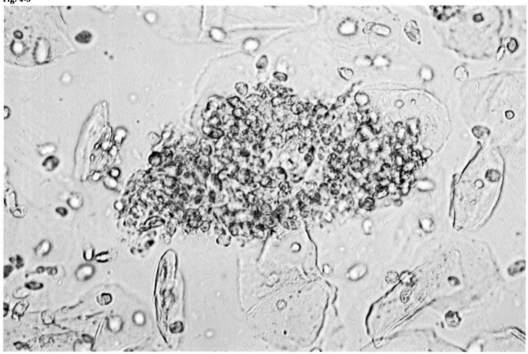

◀ **White cells, a few red cells, and bacteria.** (500×).　　**FIGURE 4-4**

◀ **Large clump of WBCs and many squamous epithelial cells.** (400×).　　**FIGURE 4-5**

Distorted white cells.　Acetic acid (2%) was added to the slide to accentuate the nuclei, thereby confirming that the distorted cells were WBCs. The reason for this distortion is unknown. (400×).　　**FIGURE 4-6**

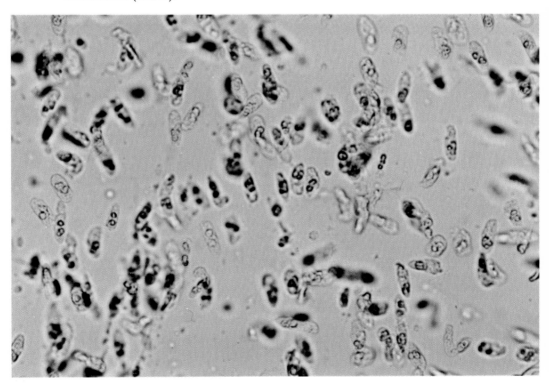

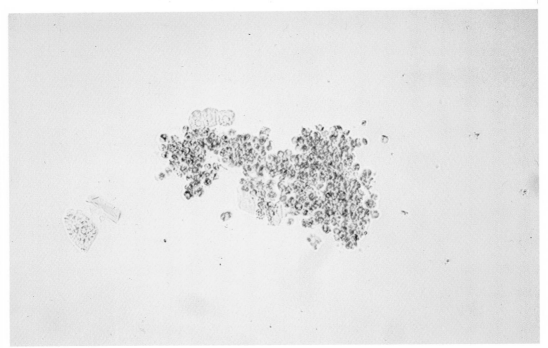

Fig. 4-7

Fig. 4-8

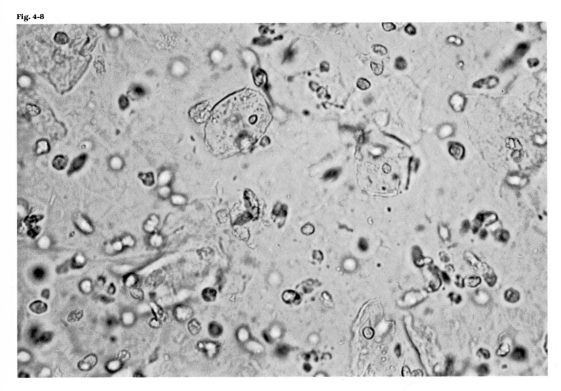

◄ **Clump of WBCs and 4 epithelial cells, all of which have been stained with bilirubin.** (200×)   **FIGURE 4-7**

◄ **White cells and squamous epithelial cells.** (400×).   **FIGURE 4-8**

Renal epithelial cells. (500×).   **FIGURE 4-9**

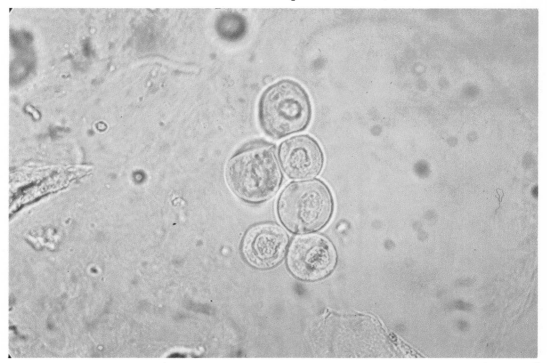

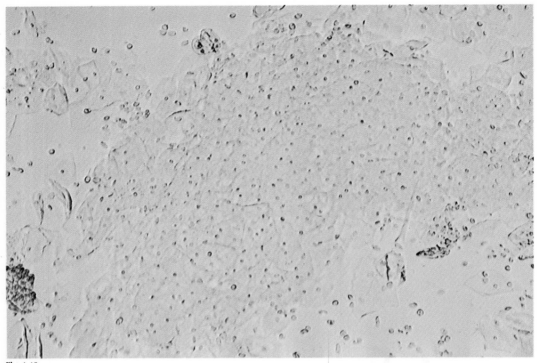

Fig. 4-10

Fig. 4-11

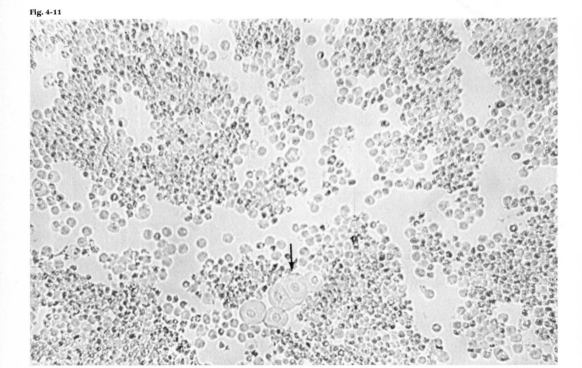

◀ **Sheet of squamous epithelial cells and WBCs.** The epithelial   **FIGURE 4-10**
cells are probably the result of vaginal contamination. (160 ×).

◀ **Numerous white cells and a few transitional epithelial cells**   **FIGURE 4-11**
(*arrow*). (200 ×).

Squamous epithelial cells and calcium oxalates. (100 ×).   **FIGURE 4-12**

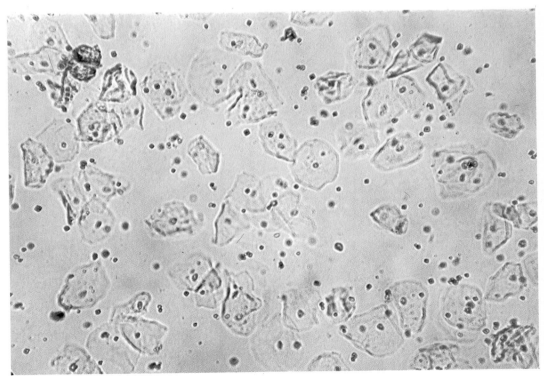

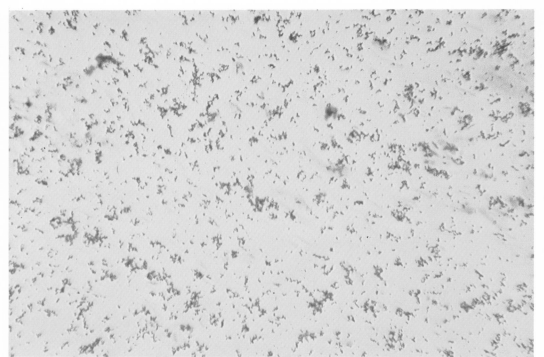

Fig. 4-13

Fig. 4-14

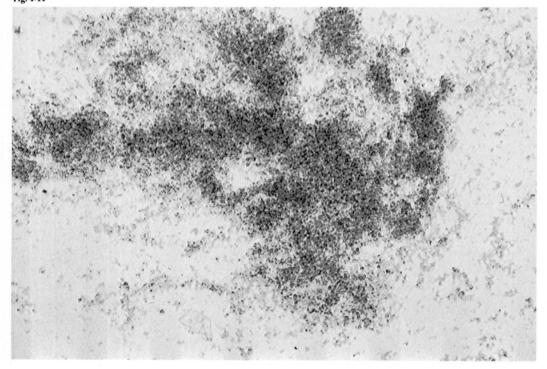

4. AN ATLAS OF URINARY SEDIMENT

◀ **Amorphous urates.** (100×).   **FIGURE 4-13**

◀ **Amorphous urates.** The urates in this field are clumped   **FIGURE 4-14**
closer together than those in Figure 4-13. Note the
characteristic color. (100×).

Uric acid crystals, diamond or rhombic form. These crystals   **FIGURE 4-15**
are very thin and are almost colorless. (400×).

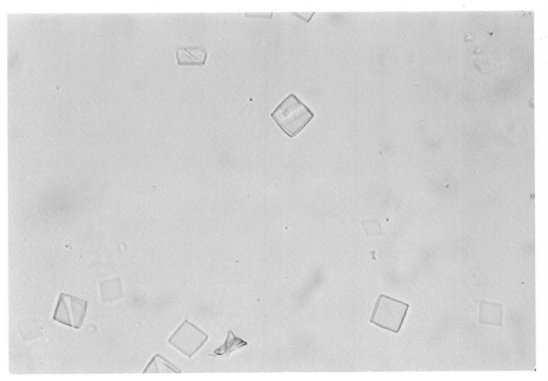

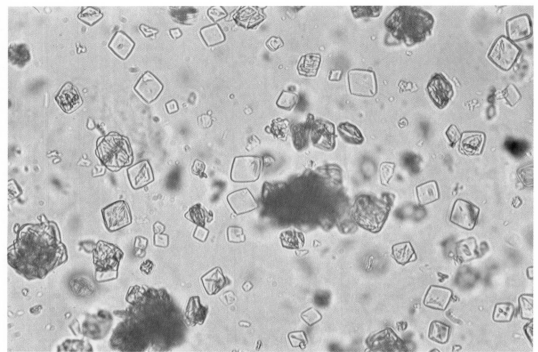

Fig. 4-16

Fig. 4-17

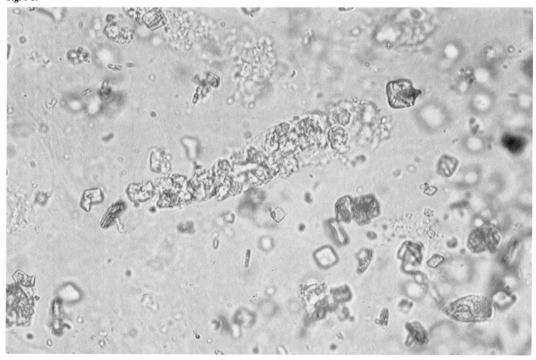

◀ **Uric acid crystals in the urine of a patient with a kidney**
stone. Note the heavy clumps of crystals that were present
even in the fresh specimen. (400×).

FIGURE 4-16

◀ **White cell cast, finely granular cast, and uric acid crystals.**
Same patient as in Figure 4-16. (400×).

FIGURE 4-17

Uric acid crystals in rosette formation. (400×).   FIGURE 4-18

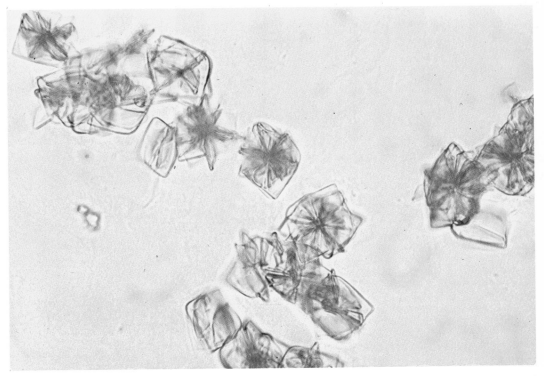

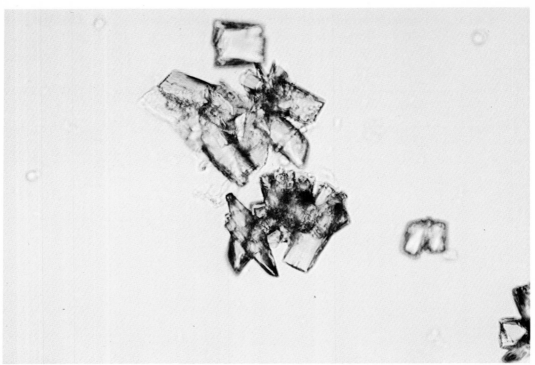

Fig. 4-19

Fig. 4-20

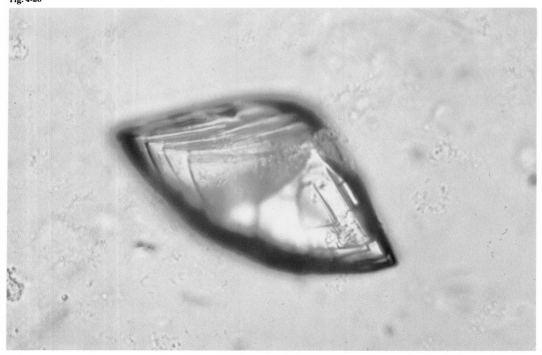

◄ **Atypical form of uric acid crystals.** (400 ×).   FIGURE 4-19

◄ **Formation of uric acid crystals.**   Note the layers. (500 ×).   FIGURE 4-20

Thick rosette formations of uric acid crystals under low power magnification. (200 ×).   FIGURE 4-21

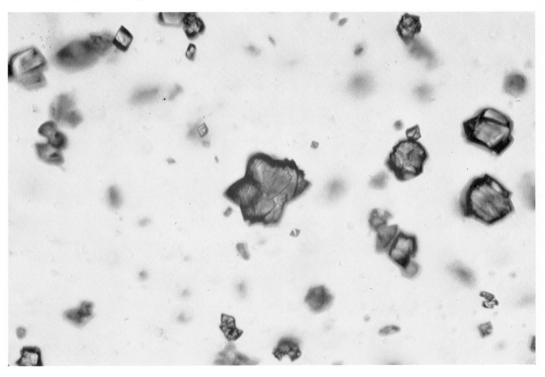

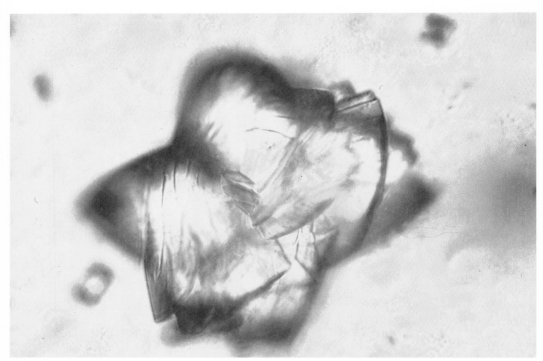

Fig. 4-22

Fig. 4-23

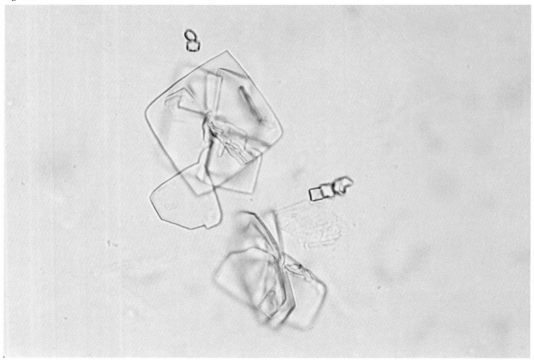

◀ **Thick rosette formation under a higher power**
magnification. Note the many layered uric acid crystals.
(500×).

FIGURE 4-22

◀ **Uric acid crystals and calcium oxalates.** (500×).

FIGURE 4-23

Polarized uric acid crystals. Note the smaller crystal. (400×).

FIGURE 4-24

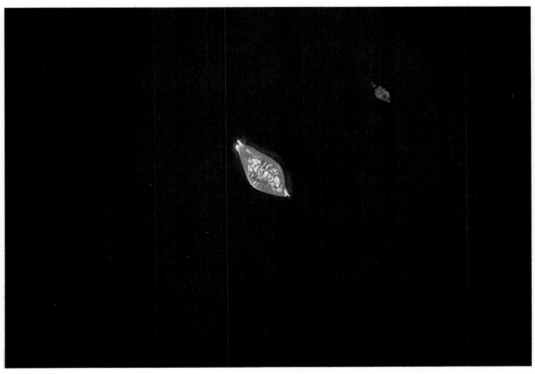

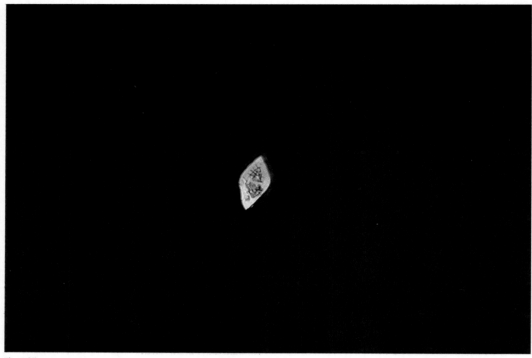

Fig. 4-25

Fig. 4-26

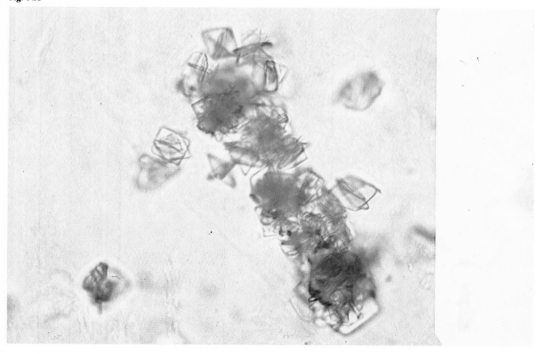

◄ **Polarized uric acid crystal.** (400×). **FIGURE 4-25**

◄ **Uric acid crystals in a pseudocast formation.** (400×). **FIGURE 4-26**

Calcium oxalate crystals. (200×). **FIGURE 4-27**

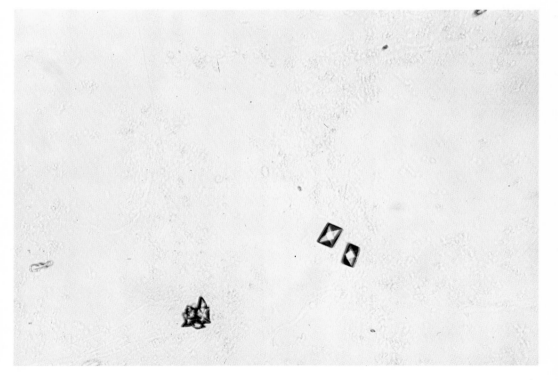

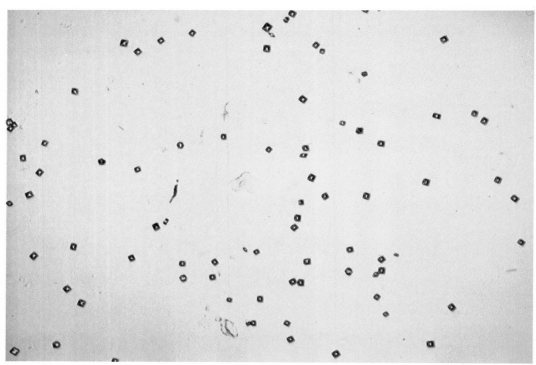

Fig. 4-28

Fig. 4-29

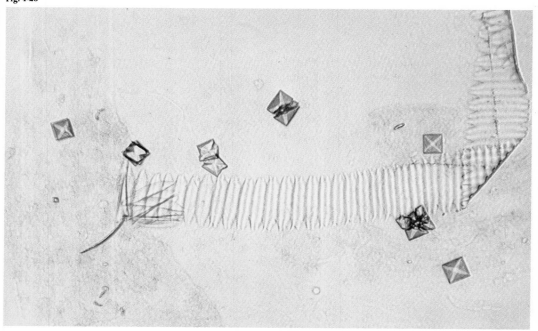

◄ **Calcium oxalate crystals.** Even under low power magnification, the characteristics of these crystals are easily recognized. (160×).

FIGURE 4-28

◄ **Calcium oxalates, amorphous urates, and a piece of debris.** Some of the crystals cracked when the coverslip was touched. (200×).

FIGURE 4-29

Calcium oxalate crystals clustered around a piece of debris. Field also contains squamous epithelial cells as well as many calcium oxalates. (100×).

FIGURE 4-30

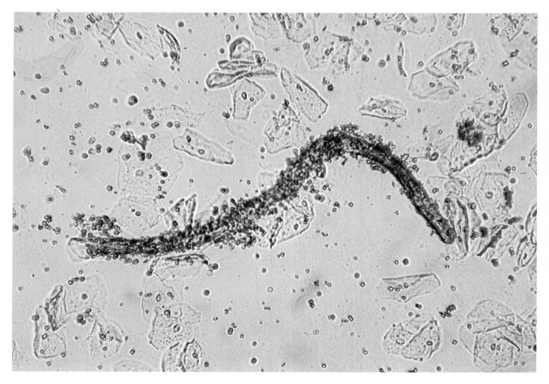

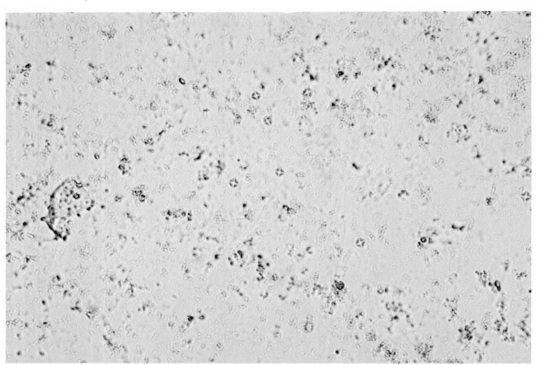

Fig. 4-31

Fig. 4-32

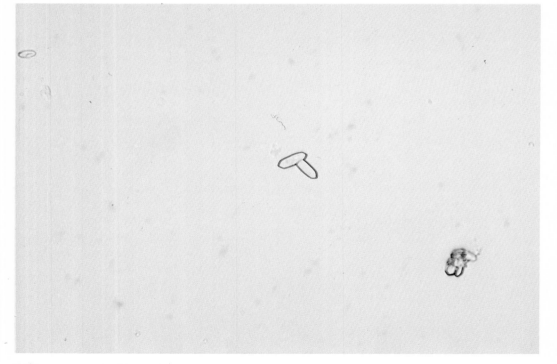

4. AN ATLAS OF URINARY SEDIMENT

◄ **Calcium oxalates and amorphous urates.** (100 ×).   **FIGURE 4-31**

◄ **Hippuric acid crystals.** (400 ×).   **FIGURE 4-32**

Sodium urate crystals. Note the square end on each   **FIGURE 4-33**
needle-like crystal. (400 ×).

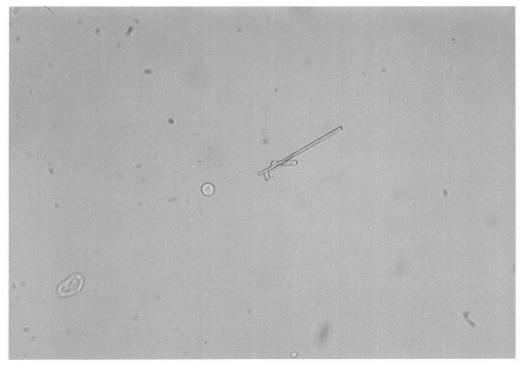

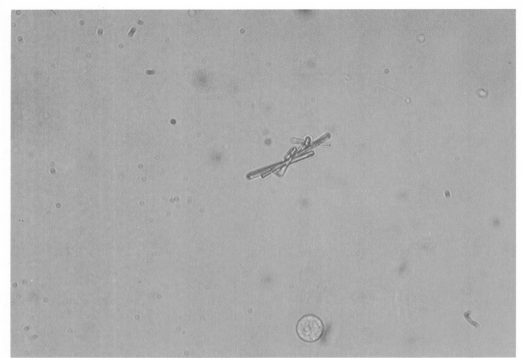

Fig. 4-34

Fig. 4-35

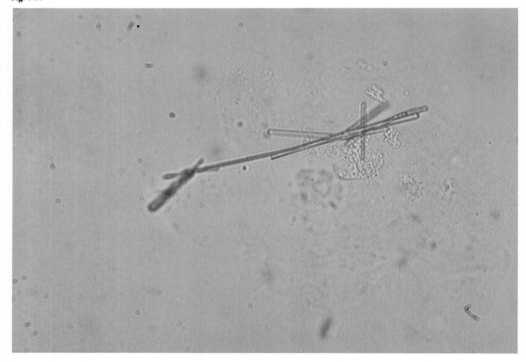

◄ **Sodium urates and a WBC.** Notice how narrow these crystals are. (400×).   **FIGURE 4-34**

◄ **Sodium urate crystals.** (400×).   **FIGURE 4-35**

Cystine crystals. (160×).   **FIGURE 4-36**

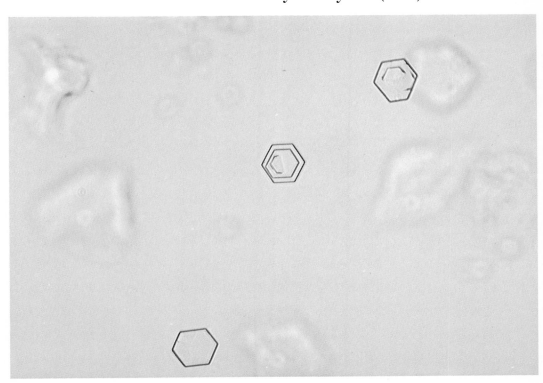

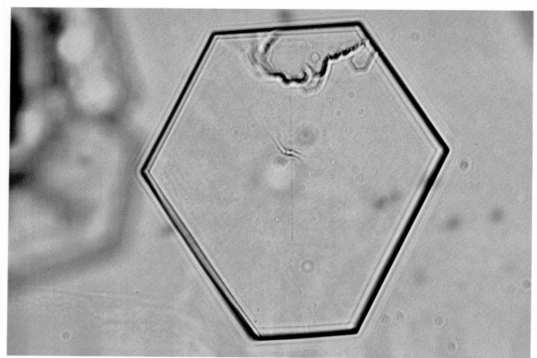

Fig. 4-37

Fig. 4-38

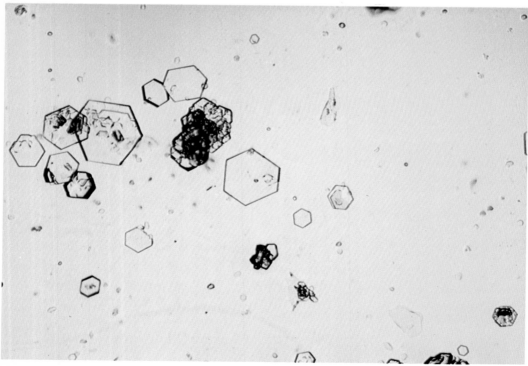

◄ **Cystine crystal with unequal sides.** $(1000 \times)$.   **FIGURE 4-37**

◄ **Cystine crystals and WBCs.** $(160 \times)$.   **FIGURE 4-38**

Cystine crystal with a layered or laminated surface. $(1000 \times)$.   **FIGURE 4-39**

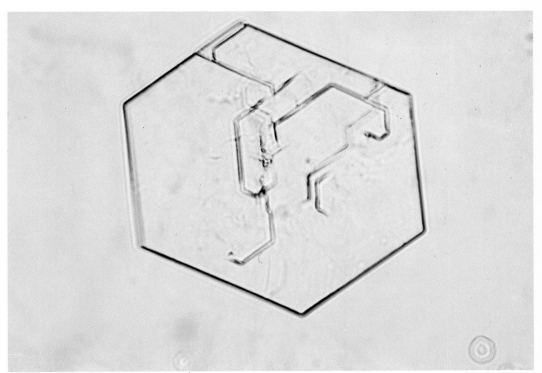

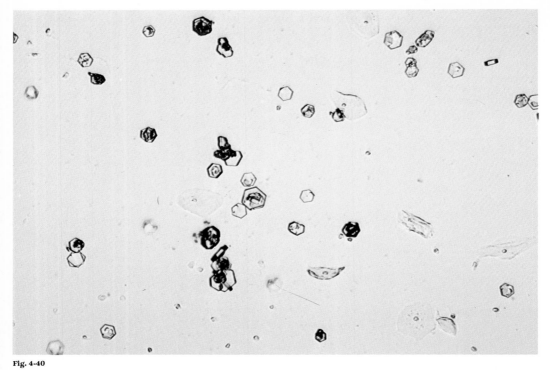

Fig. 4-40

Fig. 4-41

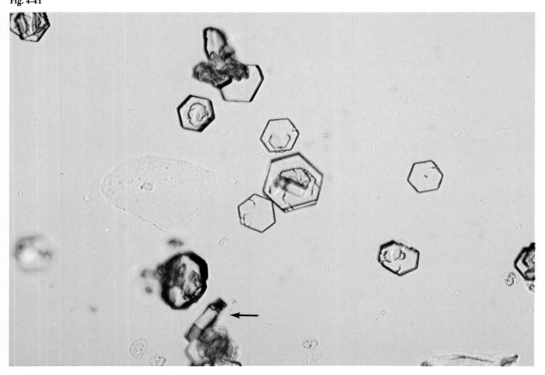

160   4. AN ATLAS OF URINARY SEDIMENT

◀ **Cystine crystals, few WBCs, and squamous epithelial cells.** **FIGURE 4-40**
(160×).

◀ **Cystine crystals and a squamous epithelial cell.** Some **FIGURE 4-41**
have laminated surfaces, and others are quite thick. The
arrow shows a thick crystal which is turned on its edge.
(400×).

Cystine crystals. Demonstration of two ways in which these **FIGURE 4-42**
crystals can occur: on top of each other, and in clusters.
(160×).

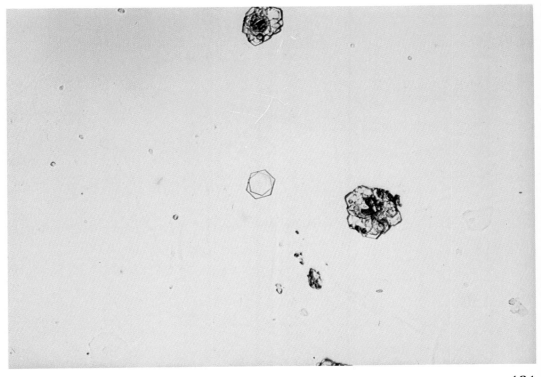

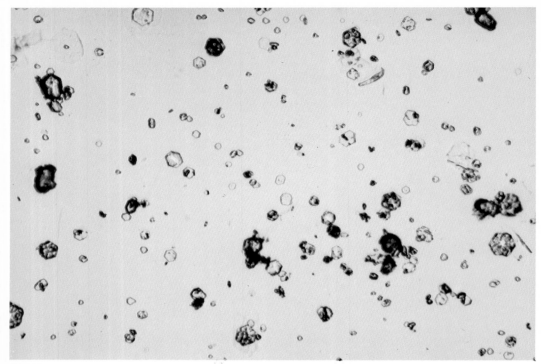

Fig. 4-43

Fig. 4-44

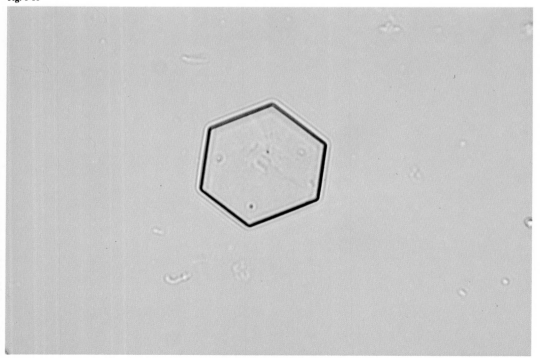

4. AN ATLAS OF URINARY SEDIMENT

◀ **Cystine crystals of various sizes.** Field also contains a few squamous epithelial cells. (160×).   **FIGURE 4-43**

◀ **Cystine crystal with a pitted surface.** (400×).   **FIGURE 4-44**

Cystine crystals in a pseudocast formation. Field also contains very small cystine crystals and epithelial cells. (160×).   **FIGURE 4-45**

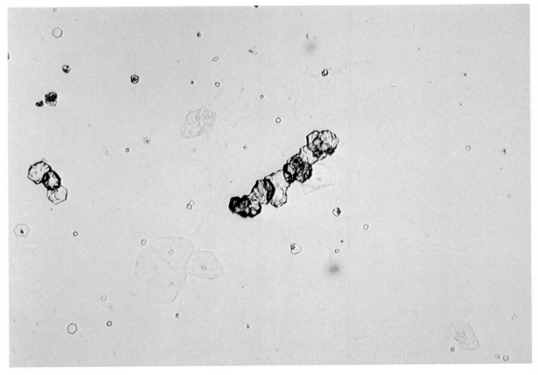

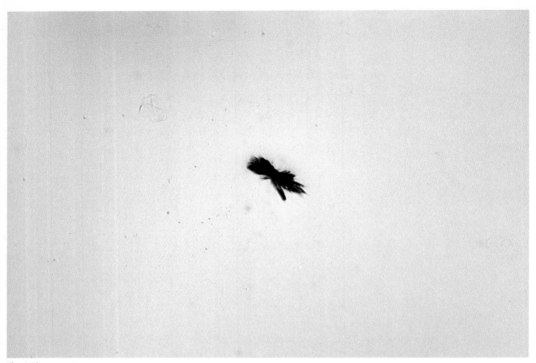

Fig. 4-46

Fig. 4-47

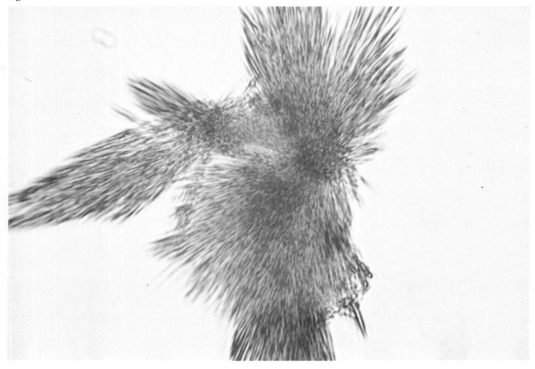

164   4. AN ATLAS OF URINARY SEDIMENT

◄ **Tyrosine crystals.**   Note how black the crystals appear under low power. (160×).   **FIGURE 4-46**

◄ **Tyrosine crystals.**   Note the fine needles. (1000×).   **FIGURE 4-47**

Tyrosine crystals. (1000×).   **FIGURE 4-48**

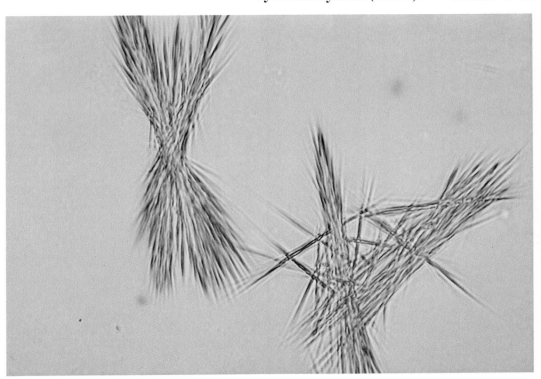

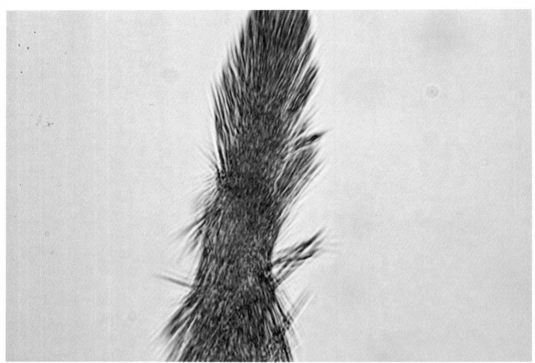

Fig. 4-49

Fig. 4-50

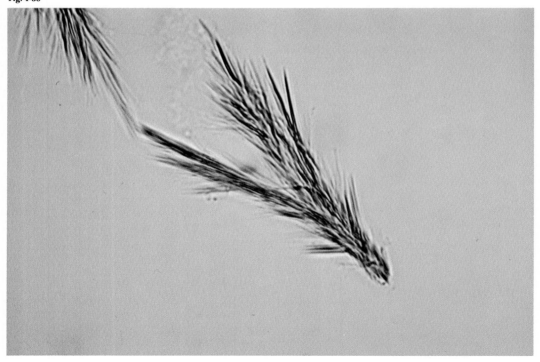

◀ **Tyrosine crystals.** Note the refractile needles. (1000×).　**FIGURE 4-49**

◀ **Tyrosine crystals.** (1000×).　**FIGURE 4-50**

X-ray dye crystals. Specific gravity was 1.070. (160×).　**FIGURE 4-51**

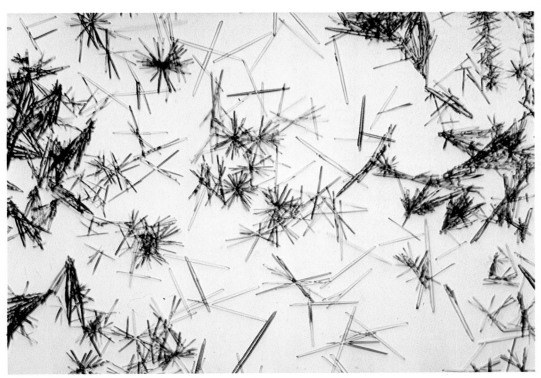

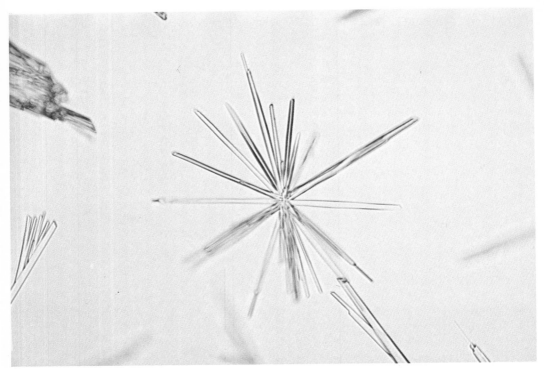

Fig. 4-52

Fig. 4-53

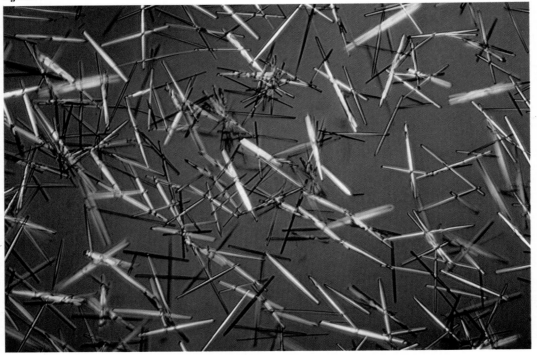

4. AN ATLAS OF URINARY SEDIMENT

◄ **X-ray dye crystals.** (400 ×).　　**FIGURE 4-52**

◄ **Polarized x-ray dye crystals.** (160 ×).　　**FIGURE 4-53**

Bilirubin crystals and bilirubin-stained WBCs and granular 　　**FIGURE 4-54**
cast. (500 ×).

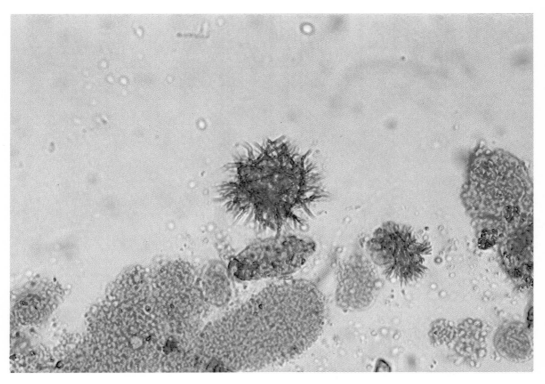

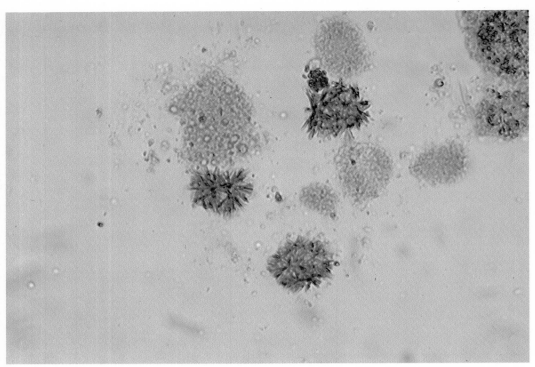

Fig. 4-55

Fig. 4-56

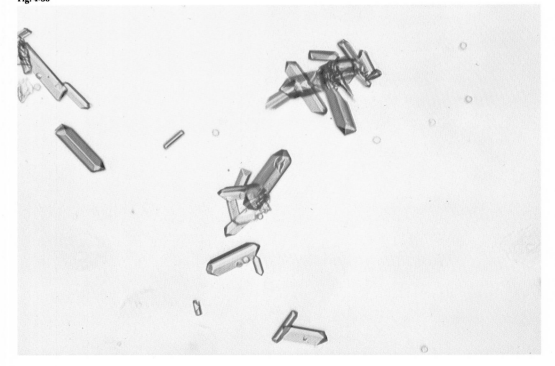

◄ **Bilirubin crystals, fat droplets, and bilirubin-stained**   **FIGURE 4-55**
   sediment. (500 ×).

◄ **Triple phosphate crystals.**   Many of these prisms are   **FIGURE 4-56**
   six-sided. (200 ×).

Triple phosphates and amorphous phosphates. (200 ×).   **FIGURE 4-57**

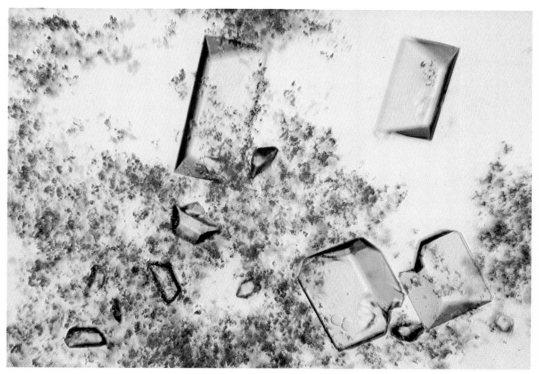

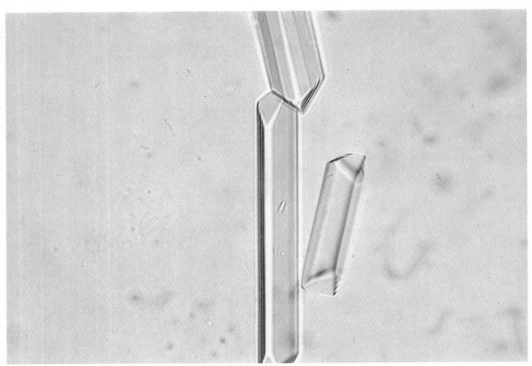

Fig. 4-58

Fig. 4-59

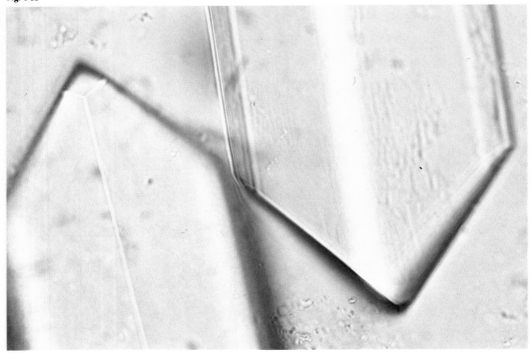

◀ **Triple phosphate crystals.** (400×). **FIGURE 4-58**

◀ **Triple phosphate crystals.** Note the sharp top edge on the **FIGURE 4-59**
left prism. (500×).

Triple phosphate crystals and amorphous phosphates. **FIGURE 4-60**
(200×).

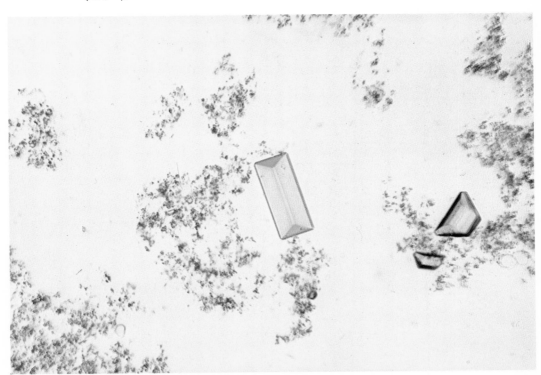

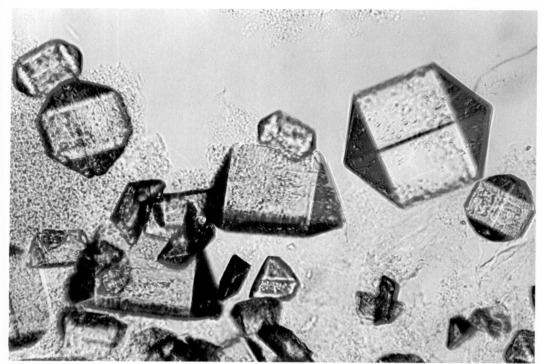

Fig. 4-61

Fig. 4-62

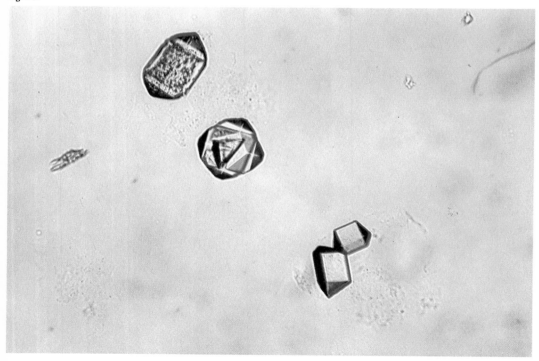

◄ **Triple phosphate crystals.** When crystals take on this grayish-black color, it usually means that they are beginning to dissolve. (200×).

FIGURE 4-61

◄ **Triple phosphate crystals.** Note the unique formation of the center crystal. (200×).

FIGURE 4-62

Triple phosphate crystal and mucous. (400×).   FIGURE 4-63

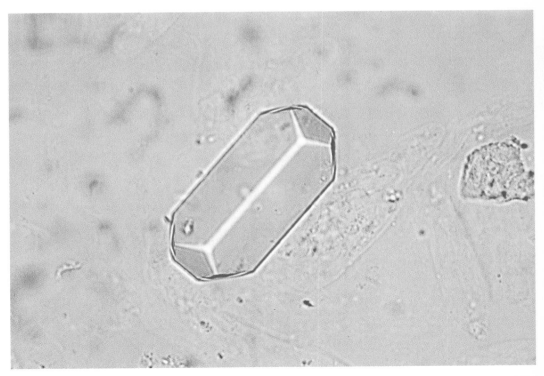

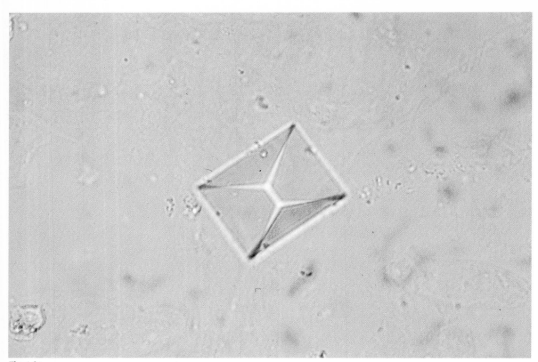

Fig. 4-64

Fig. 4-65

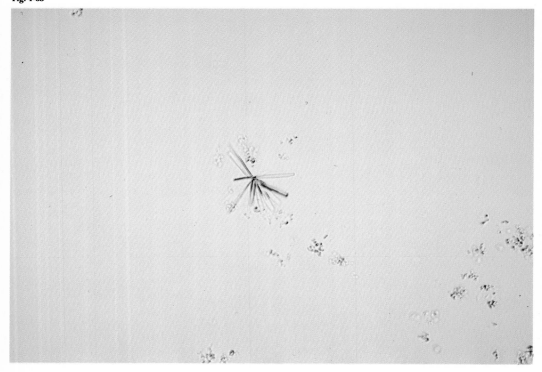

◄ **Triple phosphate crystal.** This crystal could be mistaken to be calcium oxalate, but the "X" does not cross exactly in the middle. (400×).

FIGURE 4-64

◄ **Calcium phosphate crystals.** (400×).

FIGURE 4-65

Calcium phosphate plates and amorphous phosphates. Notice the thin, granular plates. (200×).

FIGURE 4-66

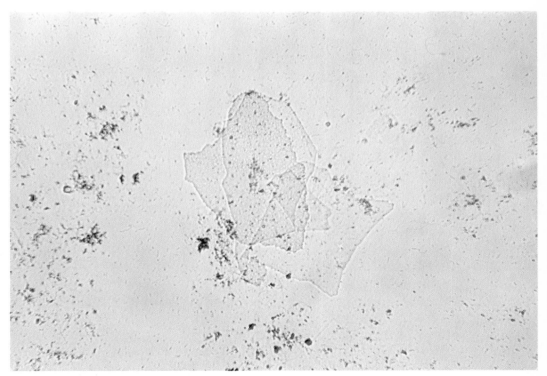

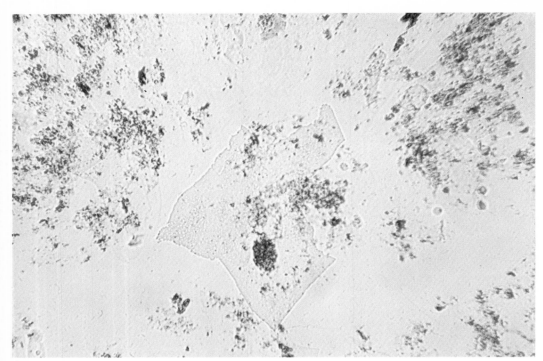

Fig. 4-67

Fig. 4-68

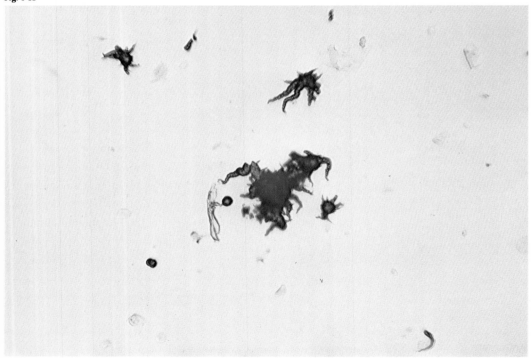

◀ **Calcium phosphate plate (or phosphate sheath) and amorphous phosphates.** (200×).   **FIGURE 4-67**

◀ **Ammonium biurate crystals.** (200×).   **FIGURE 4-68**

Ammonium biurates. (200×).   **FIGURE 4-69**

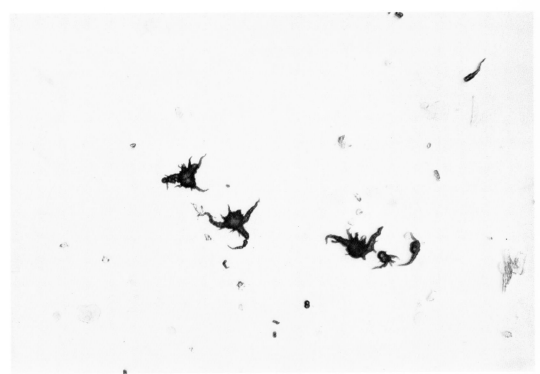

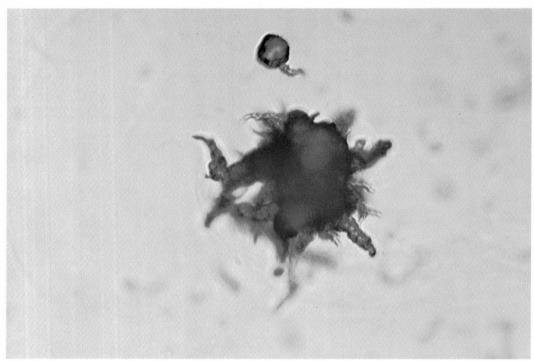

Fig. 4-70

Fig. 4-71

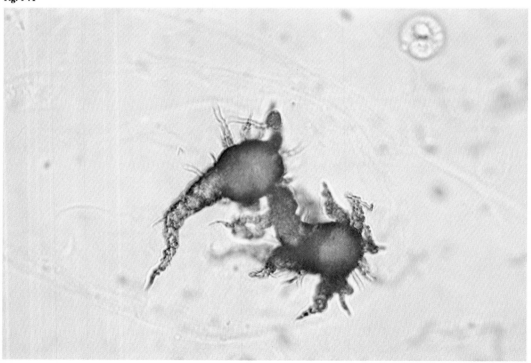

180   **4. AN ATLAS OF URINARY SEDIMENT**

Ammonium biurate crystals. $(500\times)$.   **FIGURE 4-72**

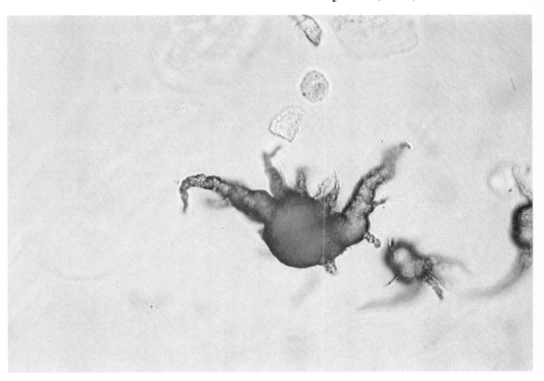

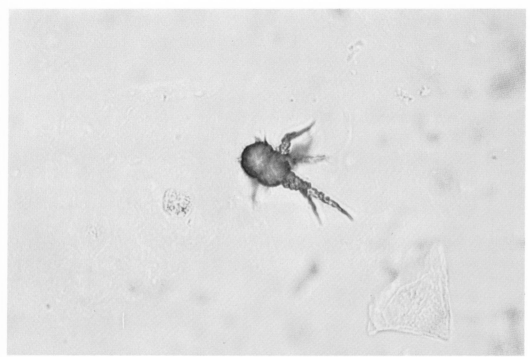

Fig. 4-73

Fig. 4-74

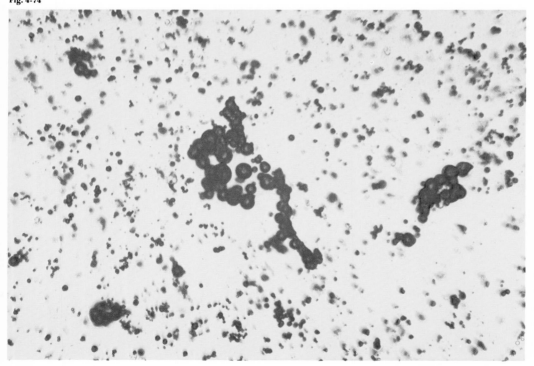

4. AN ATLAS OF URINARY SEDIMENT

◄ **Ammonium biurate crystal and a squamous epithelial cell.**   FIGURE 4-73
(500×).

◄ **Ammonium biurates.**   These are the spheroid form of the   FIGURE 4-74
crystal. (100×).

Ammonium biurates without spicules. (400×).   FIGURE 4-75

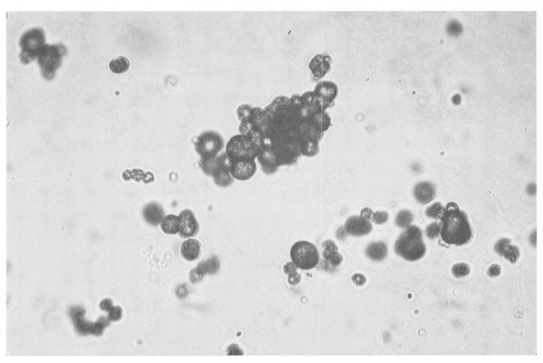

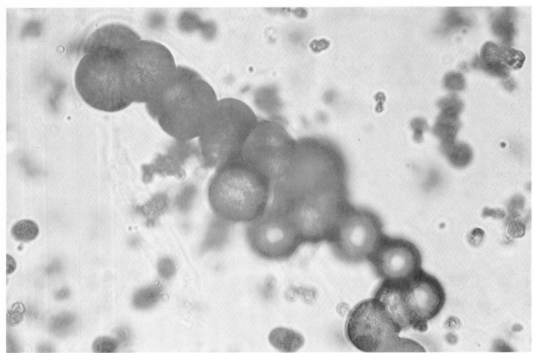

Fig. 4-76

Fig. 4-77

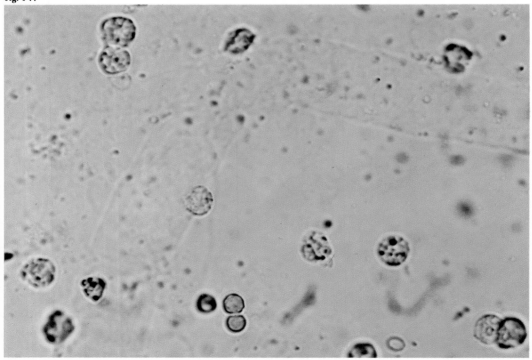

◄ **Ammonium biurate crystals, spheroid form.** (500 ×).   **FIGURE 4-76**

◄ **Hyaline cast, WBCs, 4 RBCs, and bacteria.** Can you see the   **FIGURE 4-77**
bent cast? (500 ×).

Hyaline casts. How many casts can you find? (200 ×).   **FIGURE 4-78**

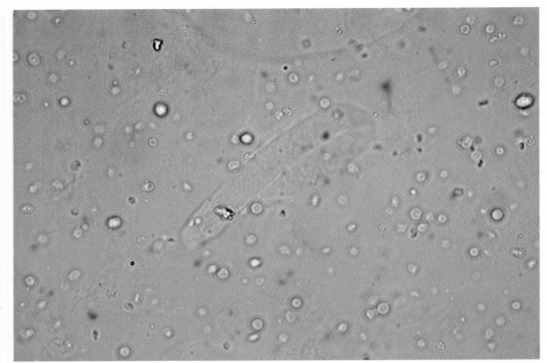

Fig. 4-79

Fig. 4-80

◄ **Hyaline cast that is bent back upon itself, and many RBCs.** Viewed with an 80A filter. (400×). **FIGURE 4-79**

◄ **Hyaline casts and many RBCs.** (100×). **FIGURE 4-80**

Hyaline casts. Viewed with an 80A filter. (400×). **FIGURE 4-81**

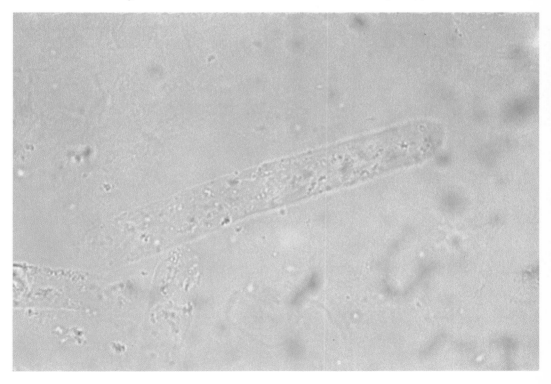

Fig. 4-82

Fig. 4-83

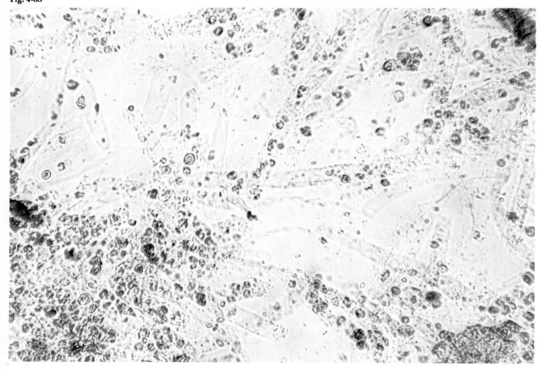

◄ **Hyaline cast.** $(160 \times)$.   **FIGURE 4-82**

◄ **Many hyaline and WBC casts, and rare red blood cell.**   **FIGURE 4-83**
    $(200 \times)$.

Hyaline cast, WBCs, RBCs, and epithelial cells. $(200 \times)$.   **FIGURE 4-84**

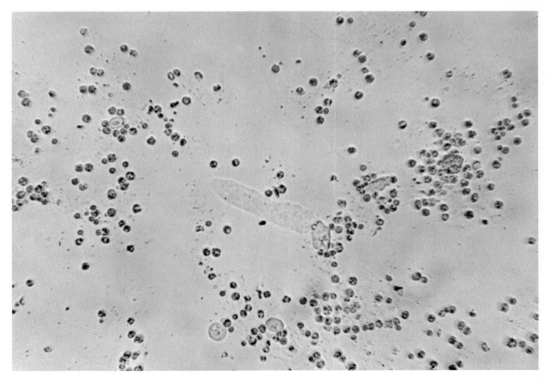

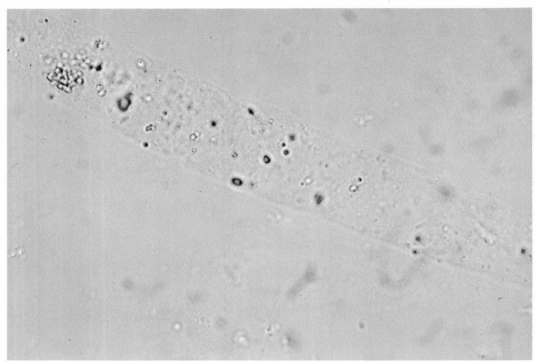

Fig. 4-85

Fig. 4-86

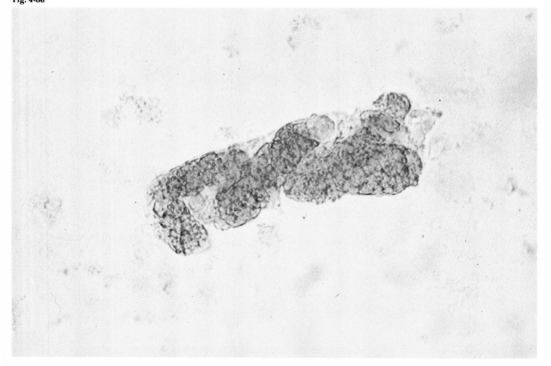

◀ **Hyaline cast with a few granular inclusions.** (500×).　　**FIGURE 4-85**

◀ **Convoluted red cell cast.** (500×).　　**FIGURE 4-86**

Red cell cast and many RBCs.　The cells in the cast are still　　**FIGURE 4-87**
intact. (160×).

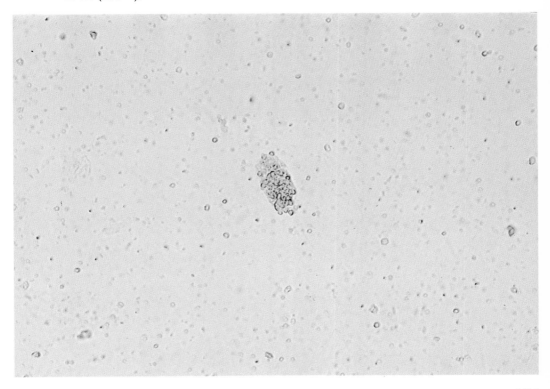

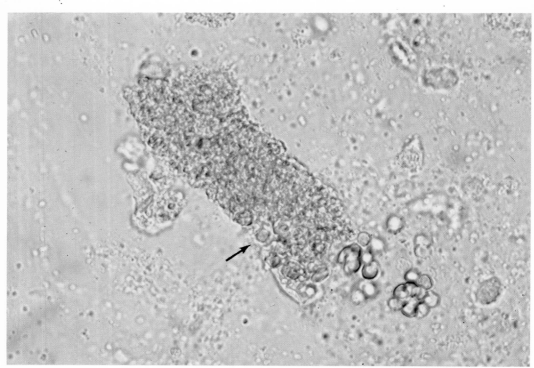

Fig. 4-88

Fig. 4-89

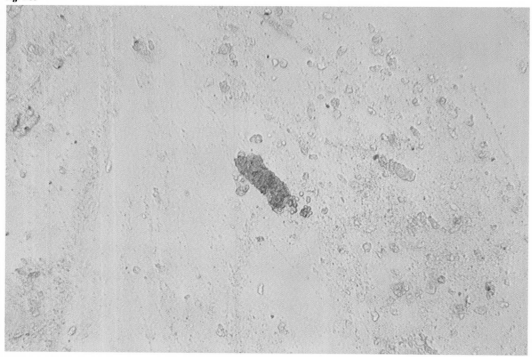

◄ **Red cell cast.** There are still some intact cells in the cast *(arrow)*, although many of the cells have begun to degenerate. (500×).

FIGURE 4-88

◄ **Red cell cast.** When the cast in Figure 4-88 is viewed under low power, the color of the cast is more prominent. (200×).

FIGURE 4-89

Red cell cast and amorphous urates. (500×).   FIGURE 4-90

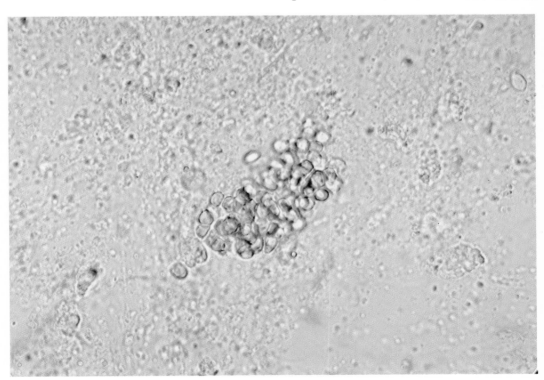

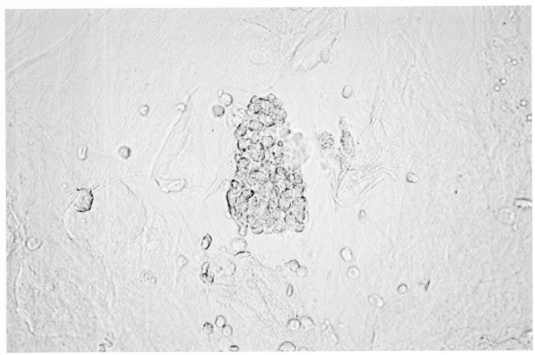

Fig. 4-91

Fig. 4-92

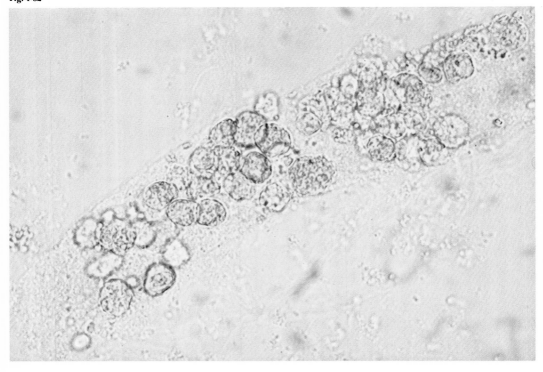

◄ **White cell cast, WBCs, squamous epithelial cells, and**   FIGURE 4-91
  mucous.   Can you see the single RBC in the cast? (400×).

◄ **White cell cast.**   The protein matrix is clearly visible. (500×).   FIGURE 4-92

White cell cast. (400×).   FIGURE 4-93

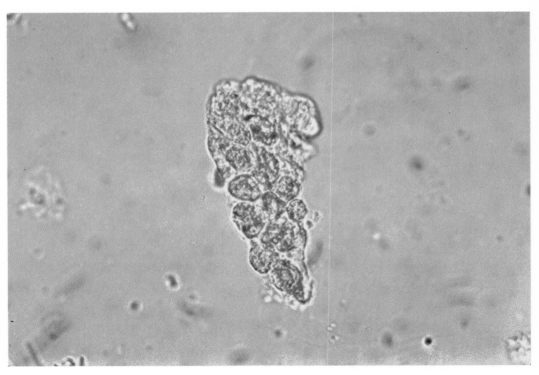

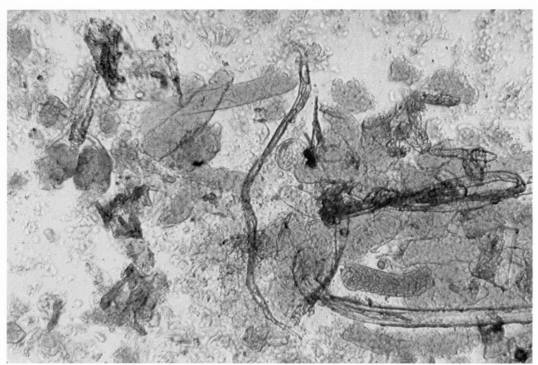

Fig. 4-94

Fig. 4-95

◀ **Bilirubin-stained casts, fibers, and sediment.** (200×). FIGURE 4-94

◀ **Mixed cast, WBCs, RBCs, and rare epithelial cell.** This cast FIGURE 4-95
contains degenerating WBCs and several RBCs, and as such,
is difficult to classify. (200×).

Bilirubin-stained WBC cast or granular cast? Bilirubin FIGURE 4-96
staining can cause problems in identifying structures, but
you can see some cell outlines. (500×).

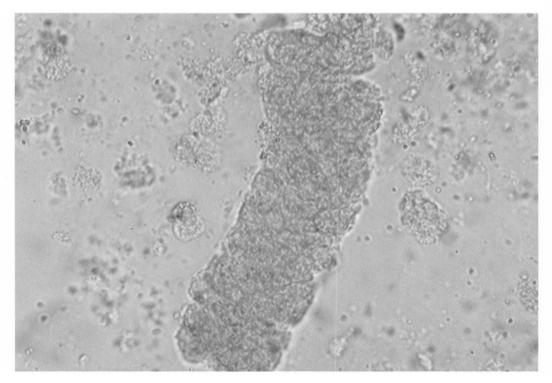

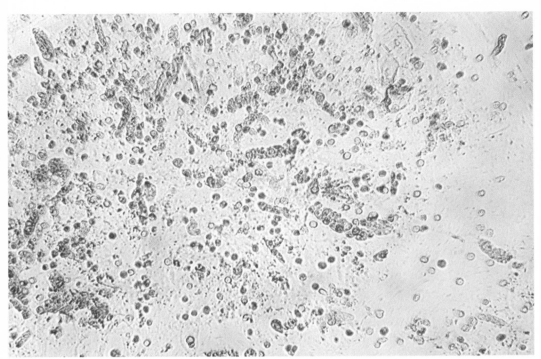

Fig. 4-97

Fig. 4-98

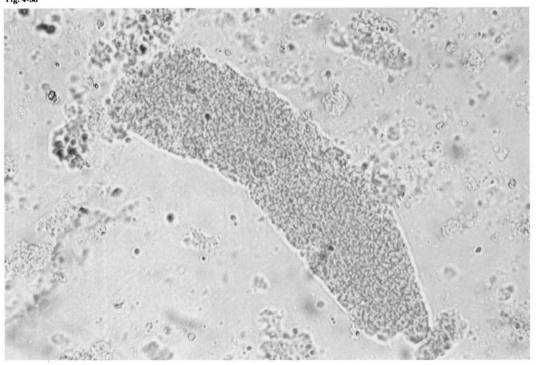

4. AN ATLAS OF URINARY SEDIMENT

◄ Many white cell casts and many WBCs. (200×).　　FIGURE 4-97

◄ Bilirubin-stained granular cast. (500×).　　FIGURE 4-98

Finely granular cast. (400×).　　FIGURE 4-99

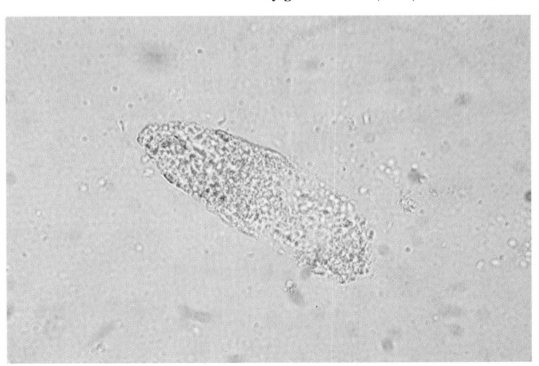

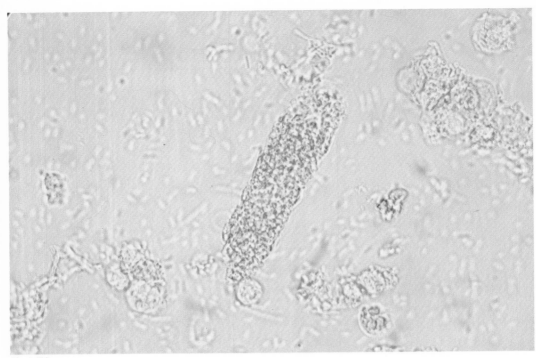

Fig. 4-100

Fig. 4-101

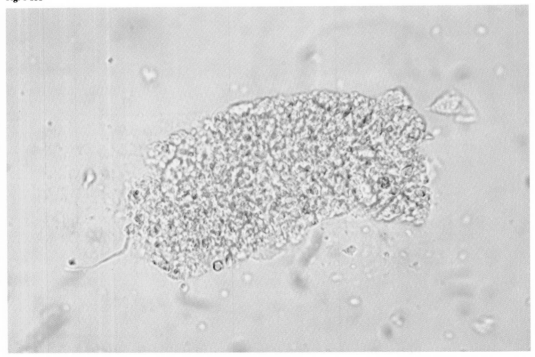

4. AN ATLAS OF URINARY SEDIMENT

◄ **Finely granular cast, WBCs, and bacteria.** (400 ×).   **FIGURE 4-100**

◄ **Broad granular cast.**   Note the width of the cast. (400 ×).   **FIGURE 4-101**

Finely granular casts, WBCs, and RBCs. (500 ×).   **FIGURE 4-102**

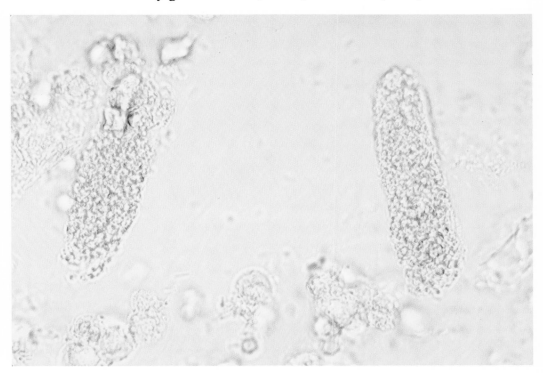

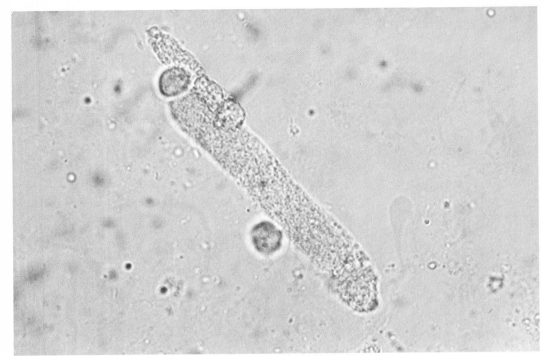

Fig. 4-103

Fig. 4-104

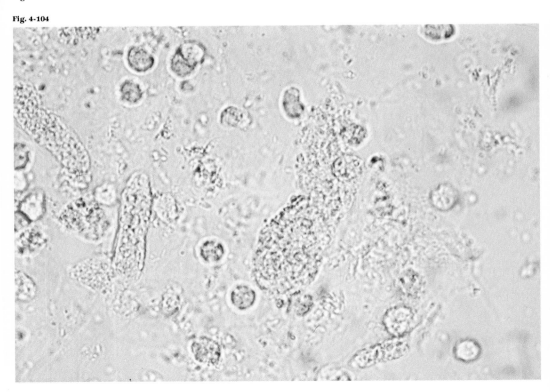

4. AN ATLAS OF URINARY SEDIMENT

◄ **Finely granular casts and WBCs.** Note the smaller cast. (500 ×). **FIGURE 4-103**

◄ **Finely granular casts and WBCs.** (400 ×). **FIGURE 4-104**

Coarsely granular cast. (500 ×). **FIGURE 4-105**

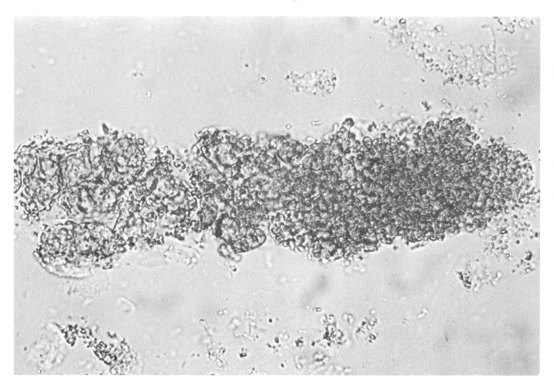

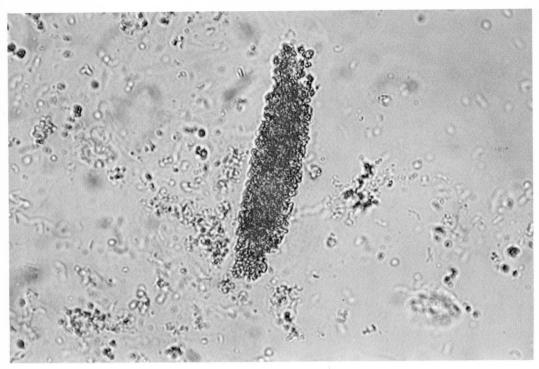

Fig. 4-106

Fig. 4-107

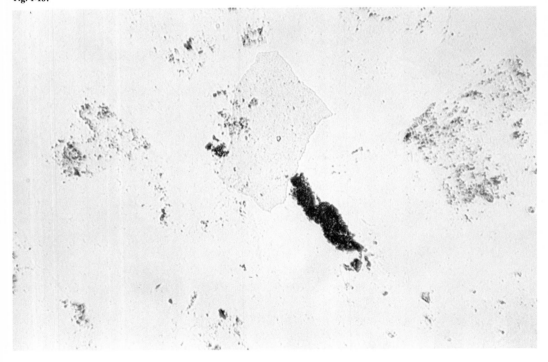

◄ **Coarsely granular cast.** (400×).   **FIGURE 4-106**

◄ **Coarsely granular cast, calcium phosphate plate, and**   **FIGURE 4-107**
   amorphous phosphates. (200×).

Coarsely granular cast. (200×).   **FIGURE 4-108**

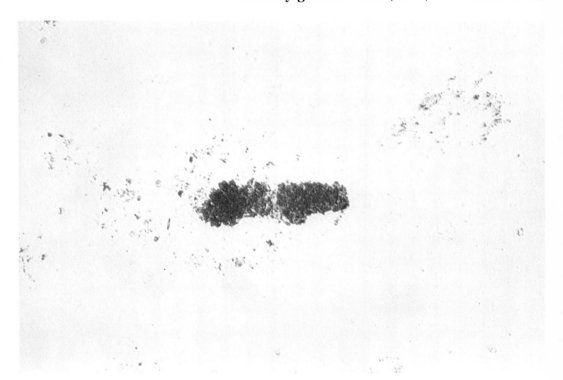

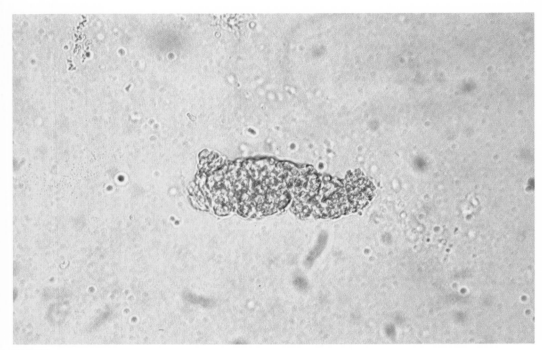

Fig. 4-109

Fig. 4-110

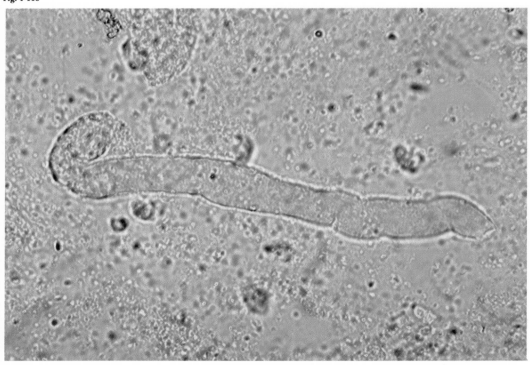

4. AN ATLAS OF URINARY SEDIMENT

◀ Granular cast. (400×).　　FIGURE 4-109

◀ **Waxy cast and amorphous urates.**　Note the indentations on the side of the cast. (500×).　　FIGURE 4-110

Bilirubin-stained waxy cast, granular cast, WBCs, and amorphous sediment.　Note the convolutions near the center of the waxy cast. (500×).　　FIGURE 4-111

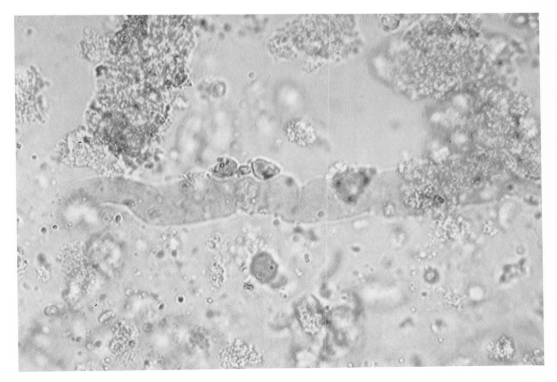

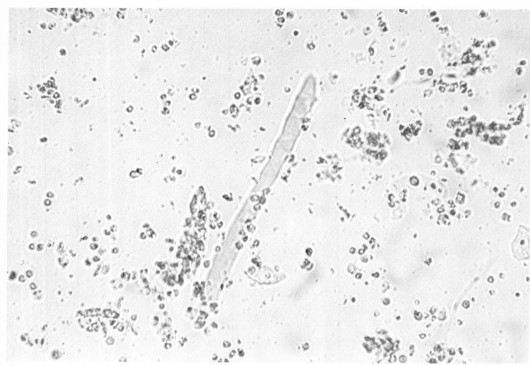

Fig. 4-112

Fig. 4-113

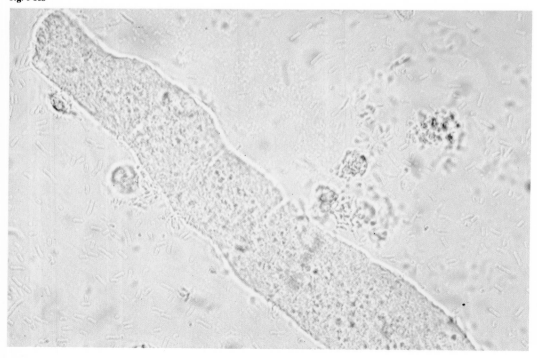

◀ **Long waxy cast, WBCs, and epithelial cells.** The surface of this cast is more refractile than that of a hyaline cast. (200×). **FIGURE 4-112**

◀ **Finely granular cast becoming a waxy cast.** Because of the typical cracks on the sides of the cast, this cast would best be classified as a waxy cast, even though the surface is still slightly granular. Note the many bacteria in the field. (500×) **FIGURE 4-113**

Convoluted waxy cast. Field also contains WBCs, rare RBC, and bacteria. (500×). **FIGURE 4-114**

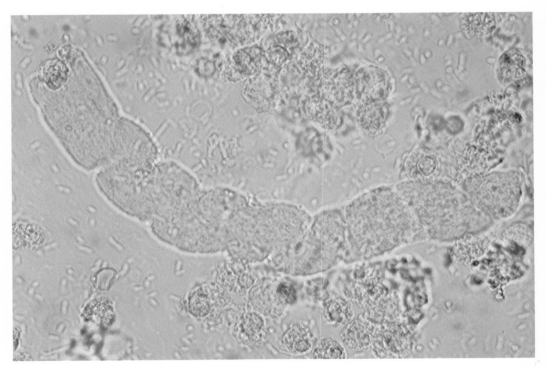

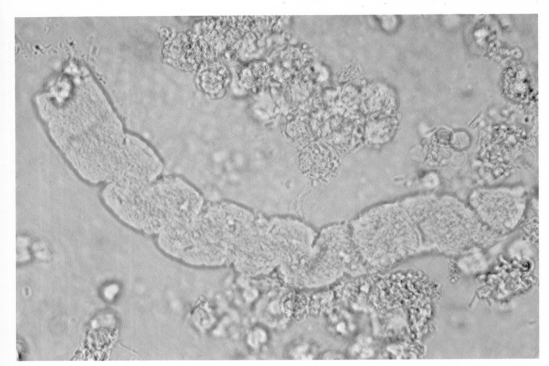

Fig. 4-115

Fig. 4-116

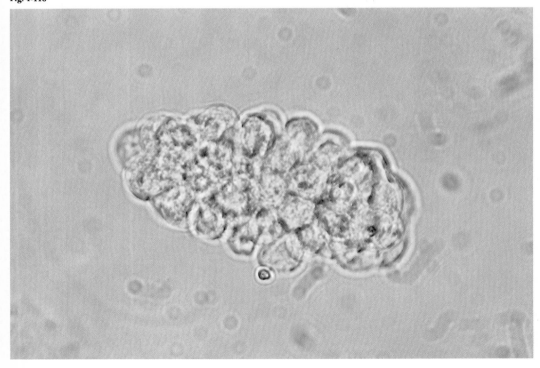

◀ **Convoluted waxy cast.** Same field as in Figure 4-114, but when the fine adjustment is turned slightly, the cast seems to develop a dark edge because of the high refractive index of the cast. (500×).

FIGURE 4-115

◀ **Epithelial cell cast.** The nuclei are visible in some of the cells. (500×).

FIGURE 4-116

Mixed cast. This cast is half hyaline and half granular. Report as "hyaline" and/or "granular," but not "mixed" cast. (400×).

FIGURE 4-117

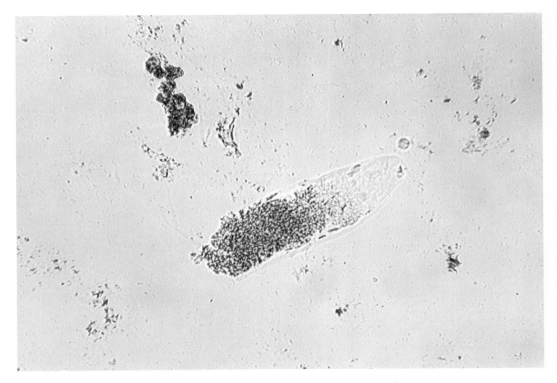

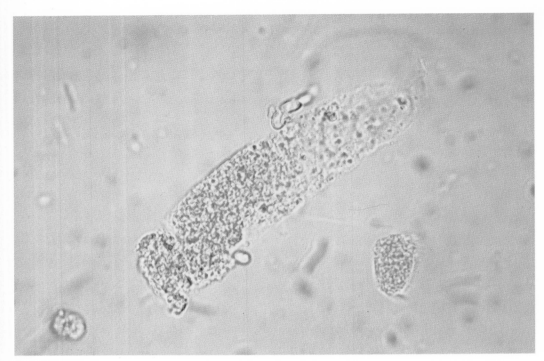

Fig. 4-118

Fig. 4-119

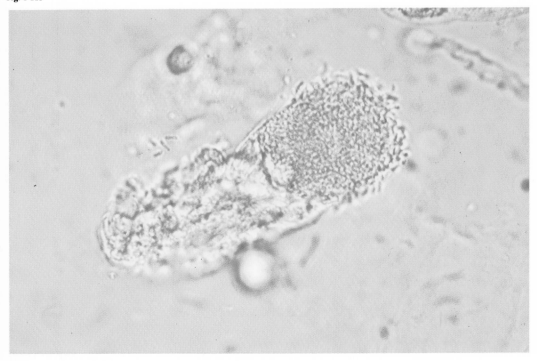

◄ **Mixed cast, yeast cells, and a WBC.** This cast is also half hyaline and half granular. (500×).   **FIGURE 4-118**

◄ **Mixed cast.** Note the bacteria in the one half of the cast. Bacterial casts are not very common. (500×).   **FIGURE 4-119**

Many casts, WBCs, RBCs, and amorphous sediment, all of which are stained with bilirubin. (200×).   **FIGURE 4-120**

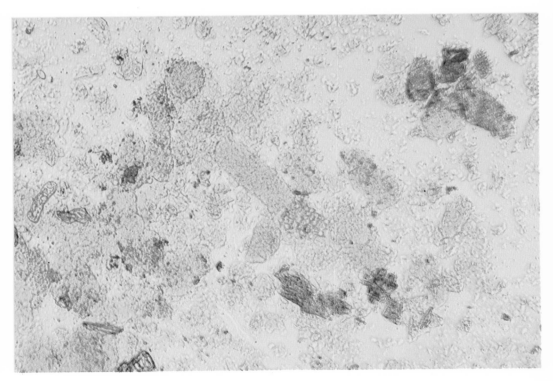

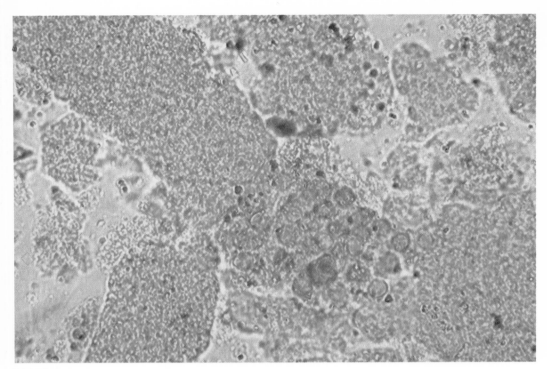

Fig. 4-121

Fig. 4-122

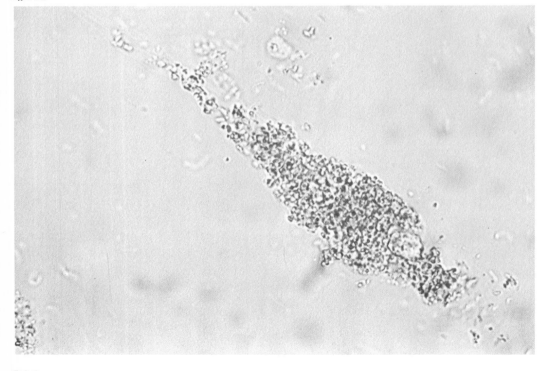

◄ **Broad, mixed granular and RBC cast, and a broad granular cast.** Same field as Figure 4-120. This specimen is from a patient with Wilson's Disease. (500 ×). **FIGURE 4-121**

◄ **Granular cylindroid.** (500 ×). **FIGURE 4-122**

Hyaline cylindroid. Note the tapering tail. (160 ×). **FIGURE 4-123**

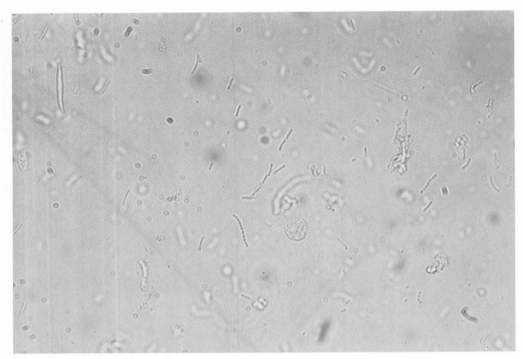

Fig. 4-124

Fig. 4-125

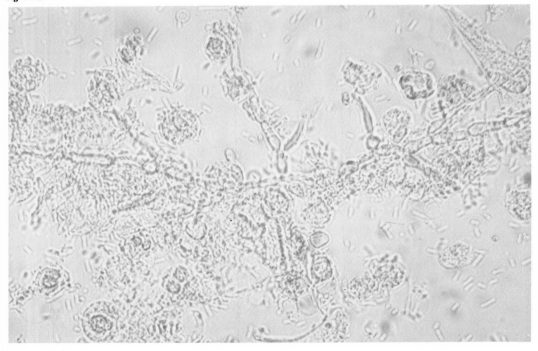

◄ **Bacteria.** Field contains rods, cocci, and chains. (500×). **FIGURE 4-124**

◄ **Yeast, WBCs, rare RBC, and bacteria.** (500×). **FIGURE 4-125**

Yeast cells. (1000×). **FIGURE 4-126**

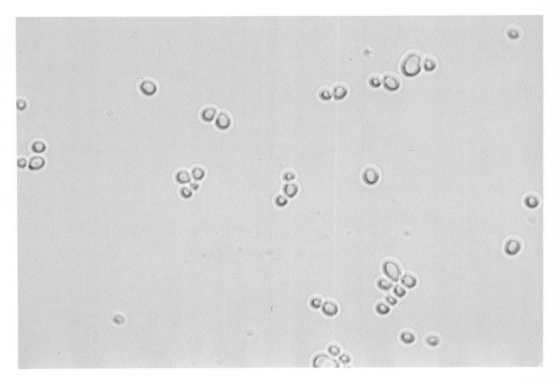

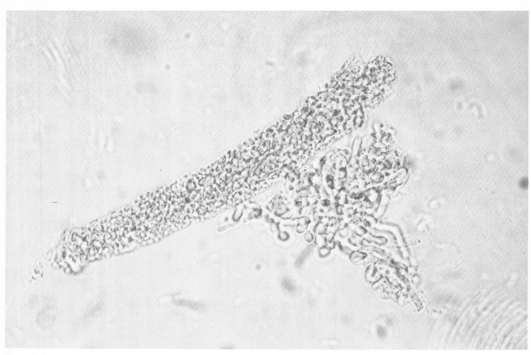

Fig. 4-127

Fig. 4-128

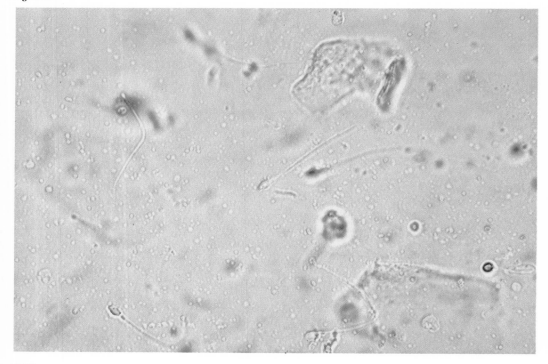

4. AN ATLAS OF URINARY SEDIMENT

◀ **Finely granular cast and yeast.** (500 ×). **FIGURE 4-127**

◀ **Sperm and epithelial cells.** (500 ×). **FIGURE 4-128**

Mucous which contains WBCs and RBCs. (200 ×). **FIGURE 4-129**

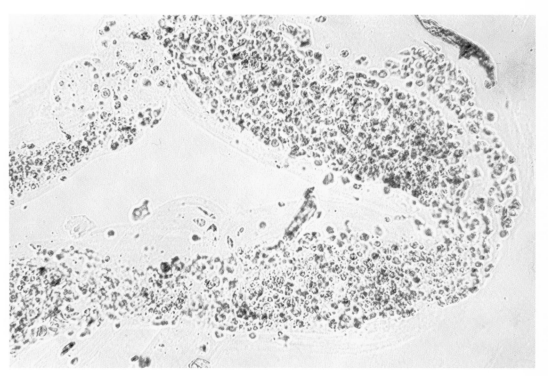

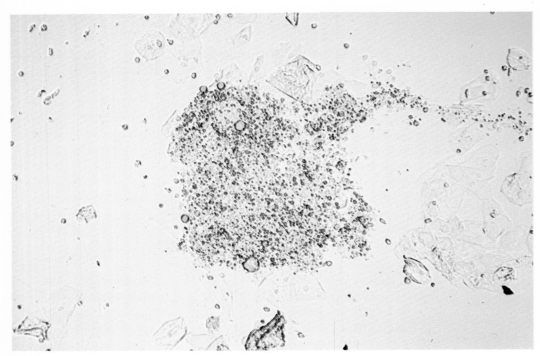

Fig. 4-130

Fig. 4-131

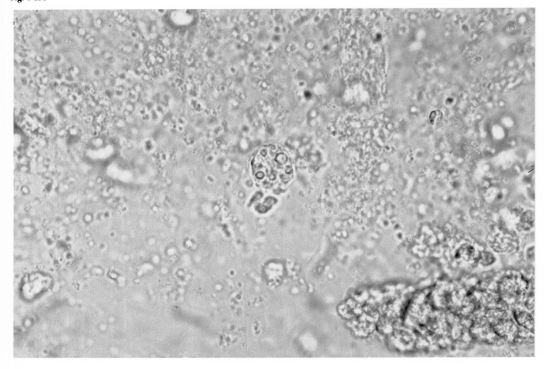

◄ **Fat droplets and epithelial cells.** (160 ×). **FIGURE 4-130**

◄ **Oval fat body, granular cast, and amorphous urates.** The **FIGURE 4-131**
oval fat body contains only a few fat droplets, thus, the
smaller size as compared to other fat bodies. (500 ×).

Oval fat body. (400 ×). **FIGURE 4-132**

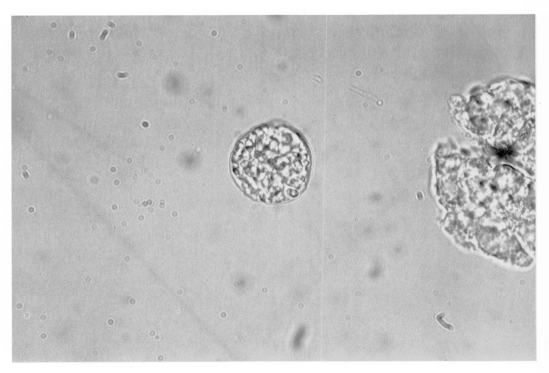

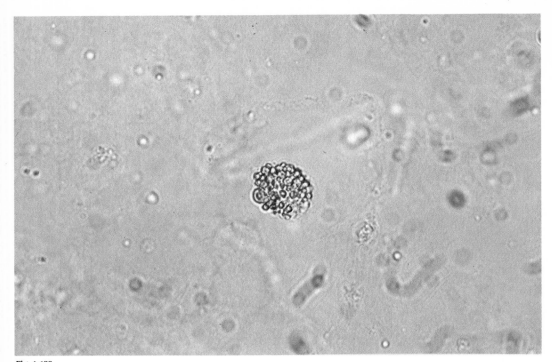

Fig. 4-133

Fig. 4-134

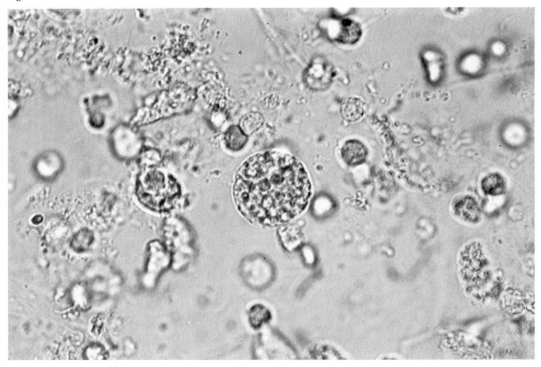

◄ **Oval fat body.** The cell is bulging with fat droplets, so the cell membrane is not visible. (500×).

FIGURE 4-133

◄ **Oval fat body and WBCs.** (500×).

FIGURE 4-134

Oval fat body. The field also contains a cell with a few small fat droplets in it (*arrow*). (400×).

FIGURE 4-135

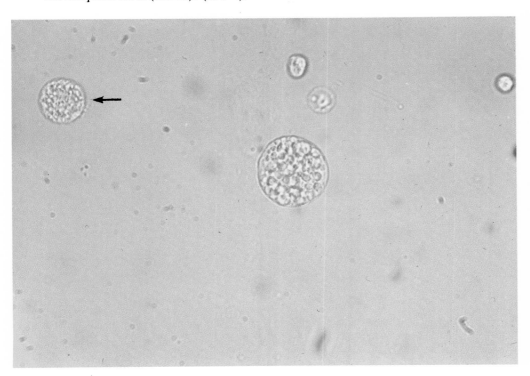

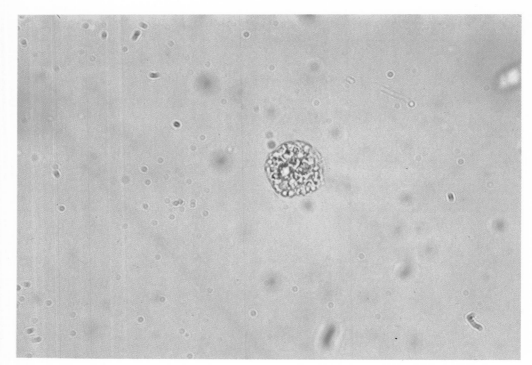

Fig. 4-136

Fig. 4-137

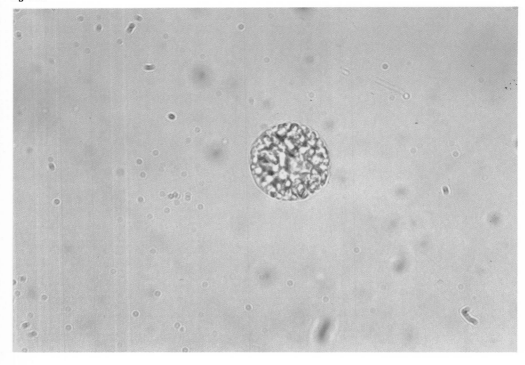

◄ **Oval fat body.** Note the various sized droplets. (400×). **FIGURE 4-136**

◄ **Oval fat body.** (400×). **FIGURE 4-137**

Starch crystals and amorphous urates. (200×). **FIGURE 4-138**

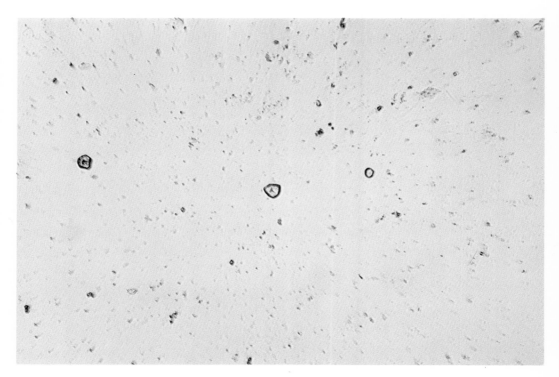

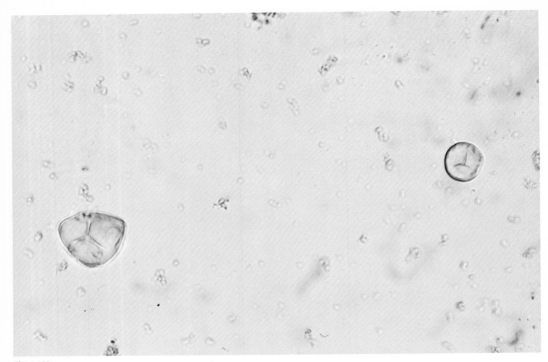

Fig. 4-139

Fig. 4-140

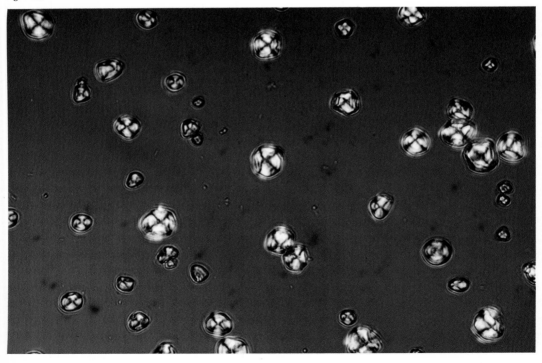

4. AN ATLAS OF URINARY SEDIMENT

◄ **Starch crystals.** Same field as in Figure 4-138. The indentation in the center of the crystal is very distinguishable. (500×). **FIGURE 4-139**

◄ **Polarized starch crystals showing the typical "Maltese-cross" formation.** (400×). **FIGURE 4-140**

Debris from a diaper. The piece of debris in the center of the field is a common contaminant. (400×). **FIGURE 4-141**

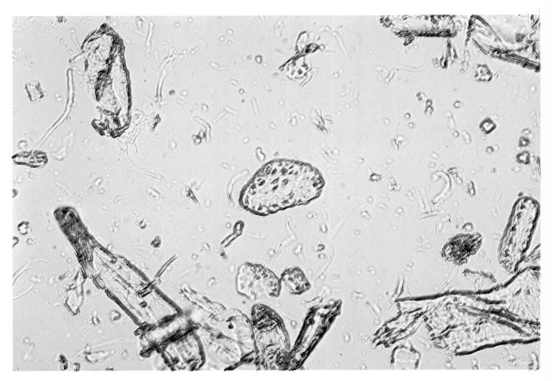

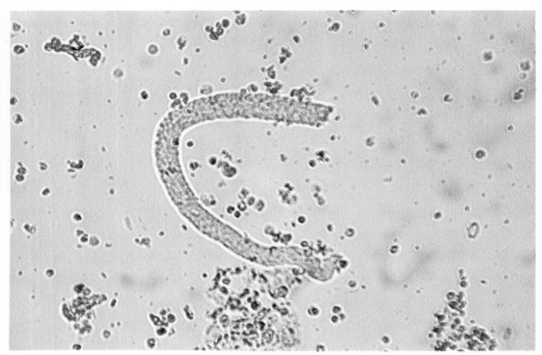

Fig. 4-142

Fig. 4-143

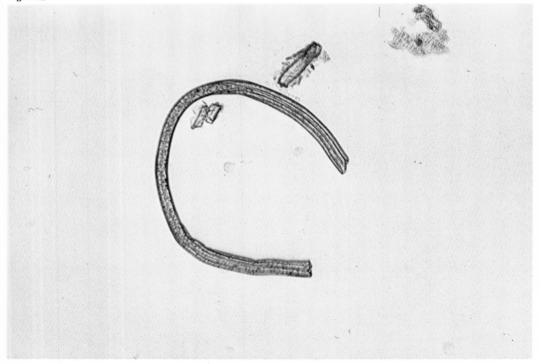

4. AN ATLAS OF URINARY SEDIMENT

◀ **Finely granular cast and WBCs.** Note the fine detail of the cast. (200×). **FIGURE 4-142**

◀ **Fiber.** Note the dark edges and the difference in texture between this piece of debris and the cast in Figure 4-142. (200×). **FIGURE 4-143**

Fiber. Note the dark edges. (400×). **FIGURE 4-144**

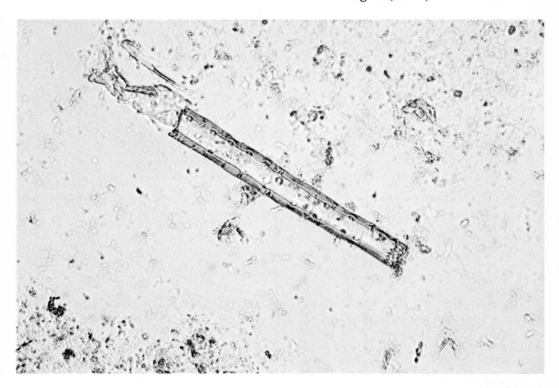

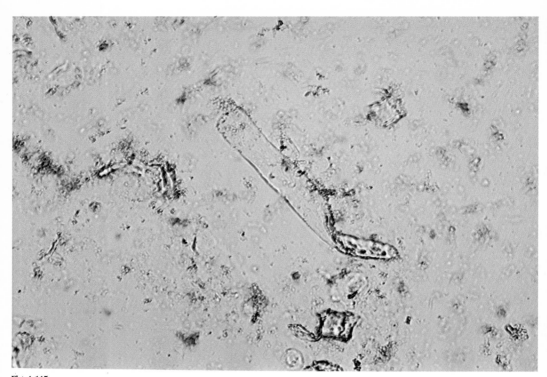

Fig. 4-145

Fig. 4-146

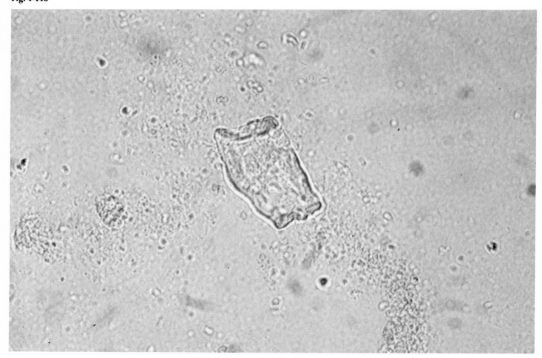

4. AN ATLAS OF URINARY SEDIMENT

◄ **Fiber.** This fiber could be confused with a waxy cast, but since part of the fiber is turned on the side, it is then noted that the structure is flat. (400×). **FIGURE 4-145**

◄ **Fiber.** Note the thick rolled edges of this fiber. (400×). **FIGURE 4-146**

Debris from a diaper. This squeezed-out specimen was worthless. Note the various types of fibers present. (200×). **FIGURE 4-147**

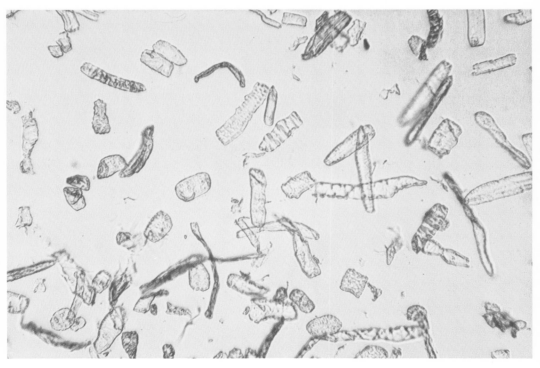

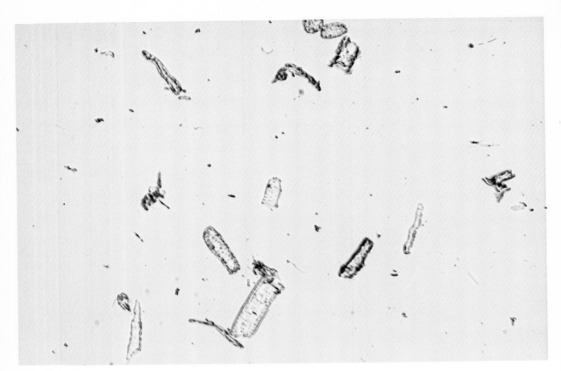

Fig. 4-148

Fig. 4-149

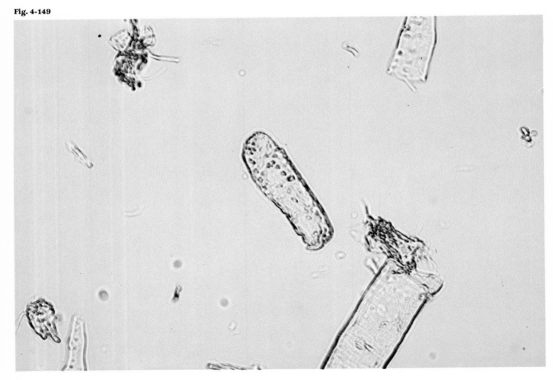

◄ **Fibers.** The striations (seen only under low power magnification) and dark edges are characteristics of these fibers. (160×).   **FIGURE 4-148**

◄ **Fibers.** Same fibers as in Figure 4-148. Note the indentations in the surface of the center fiber. (400×).   **FIGURE 4-149**

Fiber. Note the nodular indentations and nodular ends. Very common contaminant. (400×).   **FIGURE 4-150**

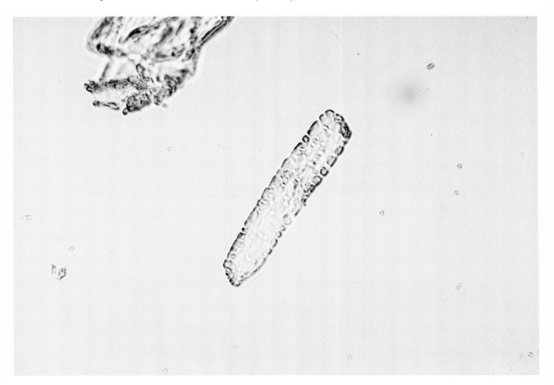

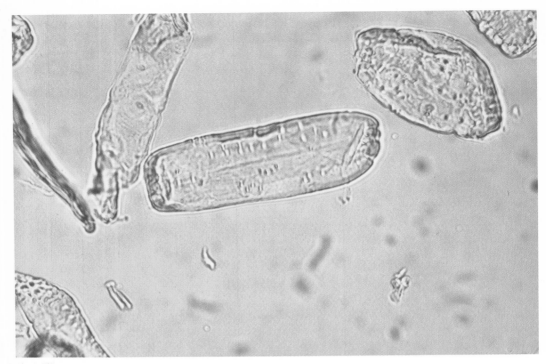

Fig. 4-151

Fig. 4-152

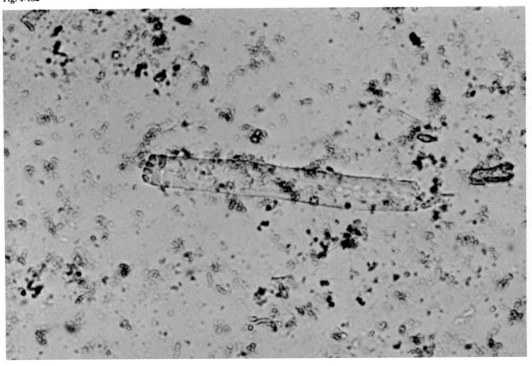

◄ **Fibers.**   The center fiber again shows a thick nodular border.   **FIGURE 4-151**
(500×).

◄ **Fiber, calcium oxalate crystals, and amorphous urates.**   **FIGURE 4-152**
Note the nodular ends on the fiber. (400×).

Fiber.   Same field as Figure 4-152, but on a different focal   **FIGURE 4-153**
plane. Changing the focus brings out the nodular
indentations on the side of the fiber. (400×).

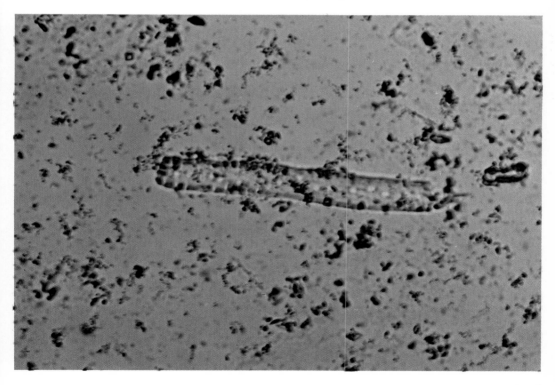

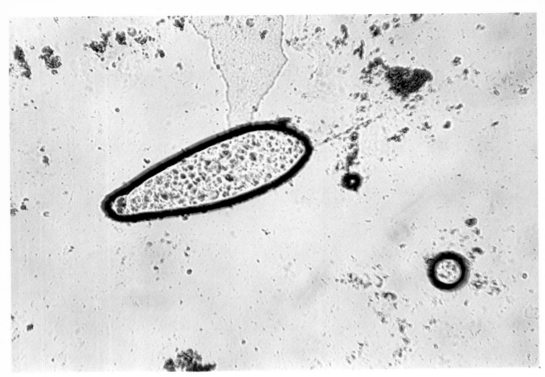

Fig. 4-154

Fig. 4-155

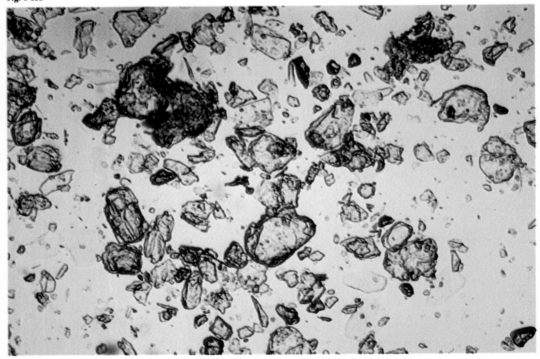

◄ **Air bubbles, phosphate plate, and amorphous phosphates.** Air bubbles can assume a variety of shapes, especially if the coverslip is moved or depressed. (200×).   **FIGURE 4-154**

◄ **Talcum powder particles and a few squamous epithelial cells.** (160×).   **FIGURE 4-155**

Pinworm ovum and WBCs. The characteristics of the pinworm ovum are easily recognized even under low power magnification. (100×).   **FIGURE 4-156**

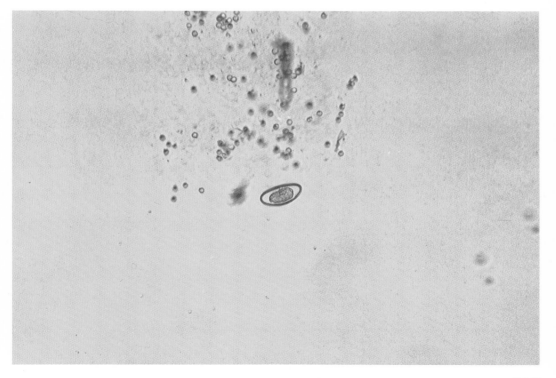

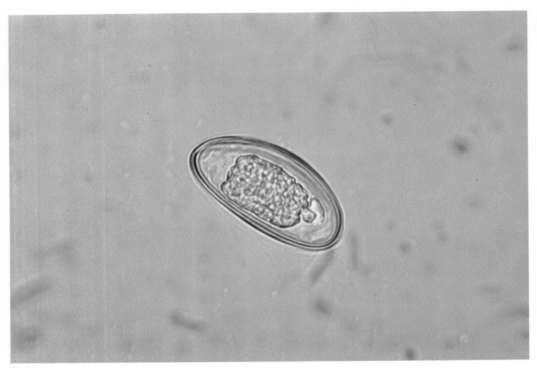

Fig. 4-157

Fig. 4-158

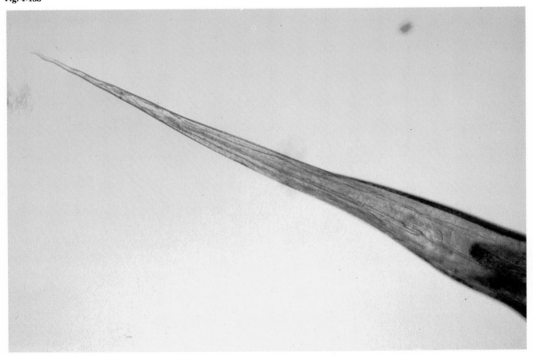

◄ *Enterobius vermicularis* or pinworm ovum. (400 ×).   **FIGURE 4-157**

◄ **Tail of the adult female pinworm.**   The tail of the female is   **FIGURE 4-158**
straight and very pointed, while the male's is curved. (40 ×).

Pinworm ovum and WBCs. (500 ×).   **FIGURE 4-159**

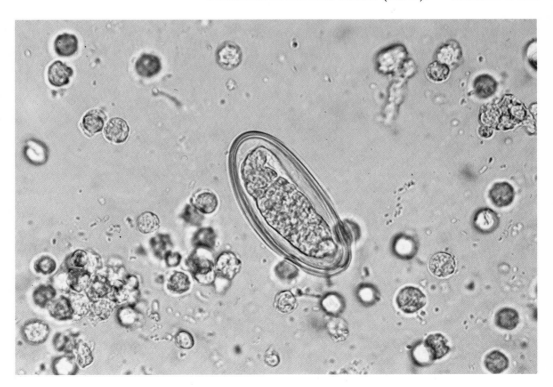

5

Special
Screening
Procedures

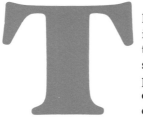his chapter contains some qualitative screening procedures which are not part of the routine urinalysis but which can be used to screen urine for the presence of certain compounds. A set of screening tests for inborn error of metabolism disorders is included because of the growing interest in the early detection and treatment of metabolic diseases. Where applicable, positive screening results should be confirmed with quantitative or specialized testing procedures and further studies.

Ascorbic Acid

High concentrations of ascorbic acid in the urine, which are found in individuals who routinely ingest large doses of vitamin C, can interfere with certain test methods for glucose, occult blood, bilirubin, and nitrite. The new dipstick procedure for leukocytes is also affected by elevated ascorbic acid levels.

There are two reagent strips, C-Stix and Stix, which can be used to detect ascorbic acid in the urine. Both dipsticks are manufactured by Ames Company, and they differ in the type of reagents as well as the levels of detection. To obtain optimum results, these dipsticks should be used on fresh urine, and the directions must be followed exactly. If interfering levels are present, the urinalysis should be repeated at least 24 hours after the last dose of vitamin C.

C-Stix

C-Stix can be used to identify urine specimens with low or no ascorbic acid content. It will also detect those levels which are associated with interference in the glucose oxidase test for glucose.

The reagent test pad contains sodium phospho-12-molybdate buffered in an acid medium. In the presence of ascorbic acid, phosphomolybdates are reduced to molybdenum blue. The dipstick is read at 10 seconds, and the intensity of the green to blue color that is produced is compared with the color chart. The color blocks represent 0, 5, 10, 20, and 40 mg of ascorbic acid/100 ml of urine.

False-positive reactions may occur if the patient is receiving gentisic acid or L-Dopa medications (Ames 1975b). Neither C-Stix nor Stix reacts with urate, creatinine, or salicylate.

Stix

Stix reagent strips are capable of detecting higher levels of ascorbic acid than the C-Stix. They cannot, however, differentiate the total absence of ascorbic acid from very low levels, because the first color block is designated 0–10 mg/dl (or normal).

The dipstick contains methylene green, neutral red, and a buffer. Ascorbic acid reduces methylene green to its leuco form and, in the presence of an inactive red background dye, the color changes from blue to purple as the concentration of ascorbic acid increases. The results are read at 60 seconds, and the values of the color blocks are: 0–10, 25, 75, and 150 mg/dl.

Unlike C-Stix, this reagent strip will not react with gentisic acid. Urines with high bilirubin concentrations or a pH greater than 7.5 may cause atypical color reactions.

Rous Test for Hemosiderin (Prussian Blue Reaction)

Hemosiderin is a yellow to brown granular pigment that is a derivative of hemoglobin (see Chapter 2). It may be found as granules that are free or in epithelial cells, and occasionally they may also be found in casts.

PROCEDURE
1. Centrifuge approximately 15 ml of urine and decant the supernatant fluid.
2. Examine the sediment for yellow-brown granules.
3. Resuspend the remaining sediment in a mixture of 5 ml of 2% potassium ferrocyanide, and 5 ml of 1% HCl.
4. Let stand for 10 minutes, centrifuge, and examine the sediment for blue hemosiderin granules.

Occasionally, the staining reaction may be delayed, so the test should not be considered to be negative until after 30 minutes.

The Ham test is another procedure that can be used to stain hemosiderin granules (White and Frankel 1965). In this procedure, a drop of sediment is placed on a glass slide, and a drop of 30% aqueous solution of ammonium sulfide is added. Mix the sediment and reagent together with an applicator stick. Examine under low power magnification for jet-black granules.

Reagent Test-Strip for Leukocytes

Chemstrip L and Chemstrip 9 (BMC) detect the presence of granulocytic leukocytes in the urine. These dipsticks contain the reagent indoxyl carboxylic acid ester and a buffer. Granulocytes contain esterases which catalyze the conversion of indoxyl carboxylic acid ester to indoxyl, which is then oxidized to form a blue color.

The test should be performed on uncentrifuged fresh urine. If the specimen has been refrigerated, it must be allowed to return to room temperature before testing. Mix the specimen thoroughly before dipping the reagent strip. The dipstick color is compared at 15 minutes, but in the presence of massive amounts of leukocytes, a blue color may develop as soon as 60 seconds after dipping.

Rarely, a positive test result may give a green color. This usually occurs when the urine has a strong yellow color from the presence of bilirubin or nitrofurantoin. Large amounts of ascorbic acid in the urine can result in falsely low reactions. The test is not affected by erythrocytes in concentrations up to $10,000/\mu l$, or by bacteria commonly present in urine (Bio-Dynamics/bmc 1979b).

As previously discussed, white cells in urine can disappear quite rapidly after voiding. However, granulocyte esterases, which are detected by the Chemstrip L, not only do not disappear, but the lysed granulocytes actually release more of their esterases in the urine, thereby giving a stronger positive test result (Gambino 1981). For this reason, if the urine has stood for a long period of time, there will no longer be a correlation between the reagent strip and the number of WBCs still present in the sediment.

Since the esterase test is not dependent on the presence of intact cells (Kusumi et al. 1981), it should prove to be a useful test, especially in conjunction with the microscopic examination.

Lignin Test for Sulfonamides

The Lignin test can be used to verify the presence of sulfa crystals in the urine. The principle of the test is that in the presence of strong acid, the arylamine group in the sulfonamide reacts with the crude cellulose or wood fiber contained in newspaper, paper towels, and matchsticks to form a yellow to orange color.

PROCEDURE
1. Place 1 or 2 drops of urine on a blank strip of newspaper or a paper towel.
2. Add a drop of 25% hydrochloric acid in the center of the moistened area.
3. The appearance of a yellow to orange color within 15 minutes indicates a positive result.

Paper of bond quality or filter paper cannot be used for this procedure (Hepler 1949). Faint shades of yellow can be produced by normal urines due to urea (place a few drops of urine on the newspaper or paper towel and see if a color develops without adding the acid). Urine from patients taking phenacetin may give a pink color, and several other substances (e.g., aniline, benzidine) give positive reactions.

Homogentisic Acid

Alkaptonuria is a rare inborn error of metabolism disease characterized by the excretion of homogentisic acid, or "alkapton," in the
urine. It is due to the congenital lack of the enzyme homogentisic
acid oxidase, which mediates an essential step in the catabolism of
phenylalanine and tyrosine. The normal metabolism of these amino
acids is shown in Figure 5-1. The absence of homogentisic acid oxidase, therefore, results in the accumulation and excretion of homogentisic acid (2,5-dihydroxyphenylacetic acid).

In adults, the disease may manifest itself as arthritis and dark
pigmentation of the cartilage (ochronosis). Infants may have darkly
stained diapers with a strong odor.

Normally, there is no homogentisic acid present in the urine.
Urine which contains homogentisic acid turns dark if allowed to
stand. Visible darkening may occur in several hours, but occasionally it may take 12–24 hours (Kachmar 1970). This darkening is the
result of the formation of polymerization products of homogentisic
acid, and the process begins at the surface of the urine and gradually
spreads throughout. If ascorbic acid is present in the urine it will interfere with this darkening process (Bradley et al. 1979).

Qualitative procedures that can be used to screen for homogentisic acid include the ferric chloride test, alkalinization, and the
film test. Positive tests should be confirmed by paper or thin-layer
chromatography.

Ferric Chloride Test

Use the same procedure and reagent for the ferric chloride test as discussed in the section on melanin in this chapter. A very deep blue
color will develop in the presence of homogentisic acid, but the color
will disappear rapidly.

**The normal metabolic pathway of phenylalanine and
tyrosine.**   **FIGURE 5-1**

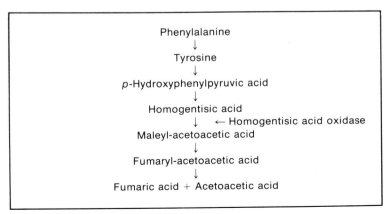

Phenylalanine
↓
Tyrosine
↓
p-Hydroxyphenylpyruvic acid
↓
Homogentisic acid
↓ ← Homogentisic acid oxidase
Maleyl-acetoacetic acid
↓
Fumaryl-acetoacetic acid
↓
Fumaric acid + Acetoacetic acid

Alkali Test

In the alkali test, the addition of an excess of 10% NaOH to the urine will produce a brown color in 1–2 minutes if homogentisic acid is present.

Film Test

In the film test, homogentisic acid acts as a developer on photographic film.

PROCEDURE
1. Alkalinize the urine by adding 0.1 N NaOH.
2. Place several drops of alkaline urine on photographic-sensitive film. (The test can be performed in full daylight.)
3. The test is positive if the film turns black.

Melanin

Melanin is a pigment which occurs normally in the skin, hair, and in the choroid of the eye. It is derived from tyrosine and is normally not present in the urine. Some patients with metastatic malignant melanoma excrete melanin or its colorless precursor, melanogen, in their urine. Upon exposure to air, melanogen is readily oxidized to the colored compound melanin, and urine that contains large quantities of melanin will become dark brown or black after standing for several hours.

Ferric Chloride Test

The ferric chloride test is based on the principle of the oxidation of the chromogen, melanogen, to the pigment, melanin. The melanin adheres to the phosphate precipitate, giving it a gray-black appearance (Beeler and Henry 1961).

REAGENT
10% Ferric Chloride—Weigh 10 g of $FeCl_3$ and q.s. to 100 ml with distilled water.

PROCEDURE
1. To approximately 5 ml of urine, add a few drops (about 10) of the 10% ferric chloride solution.
2. The development of a gray or black precipitate indicates the presence of melanin.

Bromine Test

The bromine test is based upon the same principle as the ferric chloride test, i.e., the oxidation of melanogen to melanin.

REAGENT

Bromine water—Carefully add a few drops of liquid bromine to 100 ml of distilled water. Mix. Store in a brown bottle and discard when the solution begins to lose its color.

PROCEDURE

1. Combine equal amounts of urine and bromine water.
2. The development of a yellow precipitate which gradually turns black indicates the presence of melanin.

Thormählen Test for Melanogen

In the Thormählen test, sodium nitroprusside is reduced to ferrocyanide (Prussian blue) by the reducing action of melanogen.

REAGENTS

1. Sodium nitroprusside solution—Dissolve a few crystals in 10 ml of water.
2. 10% NaOH
3. Glacial acetic acid

PROCEDURE

1. To 5 ml of urine in a test tube, add a few drops of sodium nitroprusside solution.
2. Add a few drops of 10% NaOH to make the solution alkaline, then mix.
3. The development of a deep ruby color is not specific for melanogen, since it will also be formed by both acetone and creatinine.
4. Acidify with glacial acetic acid. The *immediate* development of an azure blue color indicates the presence of melanogen. By itself, acetone results in a deeper red color, and creatinine causes a yellow color which then turns green, and finally blue (Weller 1971).

Phenylketonuria

Phenylketonuria (PKU) is an inborn error of metabolism disease characterized by the absence or deficiency of the enzyme phenylalanine hydroxylase. This liver enzyme is needed to convert phenylalanine to tyrosine in the pathway demonstrated in Figure 5-1. When the enzyme is not available, the result is an excessive accumulation of phenylalanine and its metabolites in the body fluids. Figure 5-2 shows the normal metabolites of phenylalanine which become present in abnormal concentrations in PKU (Henry 1964). Phenylketonuria, which is also called phenylpyruvic oligophrenia, gets its name

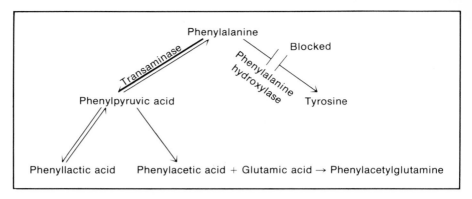

FIGURE 5-2   **Increased formation of phenylalanine metabolites resulting from the deficiency of phenylalanine hydroxylase.**

from the presence of high levels of phenylketones in the urine, especially phenylpyruvic acid.

This disease is inherited as an autosomal recessive gene, which means that both parents must be carriers of the gene, and it occurs in about 1 in 10,000 to 20,000 newborns (Frimpter 1973). If the disease is left untreated, the excessive levels of phenylalanine in the blood will cause brain damage, resulting in severe mental retardation. Other characteristics of this disease include: lighter skin and hair color than siblings, since melanin is normally formed from tyrosine; seizures; susceptibility to eczema; and the presence of the metabolite phenylacetic acid gives the urine the characteristic "musty" odor (Thomas and Howell 1973). Patients with PKU appear normal at birth but can become severely defective by age one if untreated (Stryer 1975). The treatment for phenylketonuria is a low phenylalanine diet. Because of the high frequency of PKU and the necessity for early treatment, many states now have compulsory early detection programs.

Since milk contains phenylalanine, an affected infant will show a rise in plasma phenylalanine within 1 or 2 days after the first few feedings. Urine levels of phenylalanine and phenylpyruvic acid do not become elevated until the infant is 1–6 weeks old (Bauer et al. 1968). Since the plasma phenylalanine level increases first, the required screening test is usually performed on blood before the newborn is discharged from the hospital, provided that the infant has been on milk feedings for at least 24 hours (DiSalvo and Scarborough 1978). Otherwise, the baby is tested on the first outpatient doctor visit.

The method that is most commonly used for detecting phenylalanine in the blood is the Guthrie test. The Guthrie test is a microbiological inhibition assay which uses blood that has been collected on filter paper (Guthrie and Susi 1963). The principle of the test is that the growth of *Bacillus subtilis* is inhibited by β-thienyl-alanine (which is placed in the agar), but phenylalanine, phenyl-pyruvic acid, and phenylacetic acid overcome the inhibition and allow the *Bacillus* to grow. The diameter of the area of growth around the blood-containing disk is related to the amount of phenylalanine in the blood.

Procedures which can be used to screen for phenylketones in the urine include the liquid ferric chloride test and Phenistix (Ames Co.). These procedures can be useful when doing diagnostic work-ups on families with mental retardation, since persons born before the introduction of newborn screening programs (i.e., 1965) may still remain undiagnosed (Thomas and Howell 1973). They may also be performed at various intervals (e.g., 2 weeks, 4 weeks, 6 weeks of age) on infants with negative blood results who, nonetheless, either have symptoms of the disease or are from phenylketonic families. All positive screening tests must be confirmed by blood phenylalanine determinations and clinical evaluation.

Phenistix

Phenistix test strips contain the reagents ferric ammonium sulfate, magnesium sulfate, and cyclohexylsulfamic acid. The principle of the test is that ferric ions react with phenylpyruvic acid to produce a gray-green color. The magnesium ions help to minimize interference by urinary phosphates, and the cyclohexylsulfamic acid provides the acid medium needed for the reaction.

The test strip can be dipped in urine or pressed against a wet diaper. The reagent area is read at 30 seconds and is compared with a color chart. The color blocks on the chart are designated as negative, 15, 40, and 100 mg phenylpyruvic acid/100 ml of urine. The proce-dure can detect as little as 8 mg/100 ml. The presence of any phenyl-pyruvic acid in the urine is abnormal (Ames 1978b).

Substances other than phenylpyruvic acid will react with Phenistix, resulting in various colors. Table 5-1 lists some of these substances and the corresponding color development. As noted, sa-licylates and phenothiazine metabolites give a deep purple color and, for this reason, Phenistix can be used to detect salicylate or phe-nothiazine intoxication, or to monitor whether a patient is taking prescribed medication. Large amounts of bilirubin may produce a green color. Ketones other than phenylpyruvic acid may react if they

Substances Reacting with Phenistix	TABLE 5-1
Substance	**Color**
phenylpyruvic acid	gray-green
salicylates	deep purple
phenothiazine	deep purple
p-aminosalicylate (PAS)	brownish purple
p-hydroxyphenylpyruvic acid	green, fades in seconds

are present in large quantities, as in severe ketosis. Stale ammoniacal urines may give false-negative results (Ames 1978b).

Ferric Chloride Test

The ferric chloride test uses the same principle as the reaction with Phenistix. However, this reagent reacts with a wide variety of compounds, resulting in the development of various colors (see Table 5-3). For this reason, care must be taken in interpreting the results.

REAGENTS
1. 10% Ferric chloride solution—Take 10 g of ferric chloride, dissolve and q.s. to 100 ml with distilled water. The reagent should be stored in a brown bottle in the refrigerator (Buist 1968).
2. 25% sulfuric acid

PROCEDURE
1. Place about 5 ml of fresh urine in a test tube and acidify with 1–2 drops of 25% H_2SO_4.
2. Add about 10 drops of 10% ferric chloride solution and observe the color development for 2 minutes. A dark green or blue-green color indicates the presence of phenylpyruvic or related acids. The color will *slowly* fade to yellow.

This procedure may be performed by adding the ferric chloride solution directly onto a wet diaper. It should be noted, however, that certain brands of disposable diapers have been found to give false-positive test results (Lee 1978, Kishel and Lichty 1979). Lee (1978) has therefore suggested that a positive diaper test be confirmed by the following: 1) test an unused diaper to see if there is a positive result; 2) collect another urine sample on a different brand of diaper (Pampers have not shown false-positive results); and, as always, 3) perform a blood test to confirm a positive test.

Inborn Errors of Metabolism

The term "inborn errors of metabolism" was first given by Sir Archibald Garrod in 1908 to a group of conditions that tend to run in families. These hereditary metabolic diseases are frequently inherited in an autosomal recessive manner (Buist 1968), and are usually caused by the absence or inactivity of a specific enzyme required for normal metabolic activity. The deficient enzyme may normally either produce a metabolite which is essential to the body, or it may be responsible for catalyzing the metabolism of a substance which is toxic to the body, and the accumulation of this chemical causes the disease.

Inborn error of metabolism (IEM) disorders may manifest themselves in varying degrees of severity ranging from the harmless IEM, beta-aminoisobutyric aciduria (Efron 1965), to conditions which result in early death. The most common manifestation of this type of disease, however, is mental retardation, along with other dysfunctions of the central nervous system, such as seizures, degenerative disease, or "failure to thrive" (Renuart 1966).

In metabolic diseases a variety of chemical substances are found in the urine, reflecting alterations in amino acid, carbohydrate, protein, or related metabolic pathways. At birth, the clinical and biochemical abnormalities of these disorders are usually not detectable because, prenatally, the accumulation of any abnormal metabolites is presumably cleared through the mother's circulation (Buist 1968). After birth and especially after the infant is exposed to various foods, the biochemical abnormalities become detectable usually long before there is any clinical evidence of the disease. It is, therefore, important that diagnosis be made early and treatment be initiated if possible. In this way, the pathological processes of the disease such as mental retardation may be prevented.

Aminoaciduria

The group of "metabolic-error" diseases includes the aminoacidurias, which are disorders characterized by the excretion of one or more amino acids in the urine in greater than normal quantities, or the presence of abnormal urinary amino acids or their intermediates. Efron (1965) classifies the aminoacidurias into three main groups: overflow, no-threshold, and renal-transport.

Overflow aminoacidurias are characterized by increased plasma levels of one or more amino acids, thereby resulting in their overflow into the urine. This group includes such diseases as phenylketonuria, maple-syrup urine disease, histidinemia, Oasthouse disease, tyrosinosis, and hyperglycemia.

The no-threshold aminoacidurias are not characterized by the accumulation of a very high concentration in the blood, but excessive amino acids are present in the urine because there is no normal renal mechanism for reabsorption. Diseases in which this type of aminoaciduria occur include cystathioninuria, homocystinuria, and beta-aminoisobutyric aciduria.

Renal-transport aminoacidurias are characterized by normal or low plasma concentrations of the affected amino acids, but the amino acids leak into the urine. These aminoacidurias are the result of a defective protein responsible for reabsorption in the tubule, and they can only be diagnosed by examination of the urine. Some of the diseases in this group are Hartnup disease, cystinuria, Joseph's syndrome, and glycinuria.

Aminoaciduria may also occur secondary to other diseases, such as in renal disease when damaged tubules are unable to reabsorb normal amino acids. Examples of secondary aminoaciduria include galactosemia, Wilson's disease, cystinosis, and adult Fanconi syndrome.

For a more detailed discussion of the aminoacidurias, including the defective enzymes, the affected amino acids, and other clinical manifestations of the diseases, refer to Frimpter (1973), Efron (1965), or Thomas and Howell (1973).

Screening Tests

This section includes a set of simple, rapid chemical tests which can be used to screen urine for many of the inborn error of metabolism disorders, and also to detect those patients who will require a full biochemical evaluation. Infants with such symptoms as vomiting, diarrhea, jaundice, and failure to grow may be showing signs of a metabolic disorder (Berry et al. 1968) and would, therefore, benefit from a series of screening tests. Other conditions which may be indicative of an inborn error include mental retardation, psychiatric illness, relatives of IEM patients, food intolerance, renal calculi, bone or liver disease of uncertain origin, cataracts, dislocated lenses, and speech disorders, as well as any unknown diagnosis (Buist 1968).

These tests will not detect all types of metabolic diseases, but they can detect many of those diseases which cause mental retardation or progressive systemic diseases (Buist 1968). Also, these tests are of themselves not sufficient for the diagnosis of a metabolic defect, but they are suitable for spotting suspicious cases which require careful further investigation. Laboratory resources must be available to be called upon for confirmation or rejection of the tentative diagnosis raised by a positive screening test result (Scriver 1965).

This series of tests can be performed on a random urine sample, but it should be noted that dilute urine will give false results (Stuber 1972). With the exception of the routine urinalysis and the test for reducing substances which must be performed on fresh urine, the other screening tests may be performed on urine that has been frozen for several months (Buist 1968). Specimens can then be batched and the test performed simultaneously. The tests which are included in this series include:

1. Routine urinalysis (R+M)
2. Reducing substances
3. Ferric chloride test or Phenistix
4. Cetyltrimethylammonium bromide test (CTAB) (for mucopolysaccharides)
5. Dinitrophenylhydrazine test (DNPH) (for keto-acids)
6. Cyanide–nitroprusside test (for sulfur-containing amino acids)
7. Nitrosonaphthol test (for tyrosine metabolites)
8. Ninhydrin test (for excess amino acids)

Table 5-2 lists some of the diseases which can be detected by this series of screening procedures, along with the results of some of the various tests.

Amino acid thin-layer chromatography or paper chromatography should be performed on any specimen with a positive test in the aforementioned procedures 5 through 8. Chromatography will not be discussed in this book, but one may refer to sources such as Berry et al. (1968) or Efron et al. (1964) for information on chromatographic procedures. Positive results with amino acid chromatography should, in turn, be followed up by serum amino acid studies and quantitative urine amino acid studies.

Some Diseases Detectable by Inborn Error Screening Tests TABLE 5-2

	FeCl₃	Reducing Substance	CTAB	DNPH	NaCN– Na Nitroprusside	Nitrosonaphthol	Ninhydrin (4)	Amino Acid Chromatography	Reference for *
Phenylketonuria	Green	±	−	+	−	−	±	+	
Tyrosinuria	Quick-fading green	±	−	+*	−	+	+	+	1, 4
Galactosemia	−	+	−	−	−	±*	+	+	2
Histidinemia	Olive*	−	−	±*	−	−	±	+	1
Maple-syrup urine disease	Greenish gray	−	−	+	−	−	+	+	
Lowe's syndrome	−	±*	−	+	−	−	+	+	4
Hartnup's disease	−	−	−	−?	−	−	+	+	
Wilson's disease	−	−	−	−	−	−	+	+	
Arginosuccinicaciduria	−	−	−	−?	−	−	±	+	
Hyperglycinemia	Green*	−	−	+	±	−	±	+	3
Citrullinuria	−	−	−	−	−	−	±	+	
Homocystinuria	−	−	−	−	+	−	±	+	
Cystinuria	−	−	−	−	+	−	+	+	
Hyperlysinemia	−	−	−	+	−	−	±	+	
Cystathionuria	−	−	−	−	−	−	±	+	
Fructosuria	−	+	−	±?	−	±*	−	−	2
Alcaptonuria	Transient blue-green	+	−	−	−	−	−	−	
Hurler's syndrome	−	−	+	−	−	−	−	−	
Morquio-Ullrich syndrome	−	−	+	−	−	−	−	−	
Marfan's syndrome	−	−	±	−	−	−	−	−	

Modified from Renuart (1966)
* Other references: 1 = Bradley (1971)
2 = Thomas and Howell (1973)
3 = Buist (1968)
4 = Perry et al. (1966)

A positive CTAB result should be first confirmed by repeat tests, and then followed up by a quantitative procedure for mucopolysaccharides.

Specimens having a positive test for reducing substances but a negative test for glucose should first be repeated, and then checked for interfering substances such as ascorbic acid. Confirmed positive tests should be evaluated by either chromatography or fermentation studies to determine if a non-glucose sugar is present. This procedure is important for the detection of carbohydrate disorders such as galactosemia. As with many of the IEM disorders, the early detection and treatment of galactosemia (treatment = lactose- and galactose-free diet [no milk]) can lessen or remove all symptoms of the disease.

Urines that have been frozen should be thawed out and mixed well before testing. If the urine is not clear, it should be centrifuged before performing the DNPH and CTAB tests.

Urine specimens that have been wrung out of a wet diaper, or contaminated with feces, or have been allowed to stand at room temperature for hours are unsuitable and should not be tested (Perry et al. 1966). Studies by Vidler and Wilcken (1978) show that heavy bacterial contamination of the urine may be a source of false-negative and false-positive screening tests, so care must be taken in collecting the urine specimen.

FERRIC CHLORIDE TEST

The ferric chloride test is the same as the one discussed in the section on phenylketonuria, but the volume of urine is decreased, so that the series of tests can be performed on the smallest amount of urine. This test will detect classic phenylketonuria, but the test is quite non-specific and yields a variety of color changes with certain substances. The Phenistix may be substituted for the ferric chloride test.

REAGENTS

1. 10% $FeCl_3$ solution—Take 10 g of ferric chloride, dissolve and q.s. to 100 ml with distilled water. The reagent should be stored in a brown bottle in the refrigerator.
2. 25% sulfuric acid

PROCEDURE

1. Place 1–2 ml of urine in a test tube and acidify with 1 drop of 25% H_2SO_4.
2. Add the $FeCl_3$ solution drop by drop and observe the color development for 2 minutes. A dark green or blue-green color that *slowly* fades back to yellow indicates the presence of phenylpyruvic or related acids. Refer to Table 5-3 for some of the other substances which react with ferric chloride and the color that is produced.

Substance	Color Produced
Phenylpyruvic acid	Green or blue-green eventually fading to yellow
p-Hydroxyphenylpyruvic acid	Green, fades in seconds
Homogentisic acid	Blue or green, fades slowly
Imidazolepyruvic acid	Green or blue-green
Xanthurenic acid	Deep green, later brown
Bilirubin	Blue-green
Maple-syrup urine disease	Gray with a green tinge
Melanin	Gray precipitate, turning black
3-Hydroxanthranilic acid	Immediate deep brown
Vanillic acid	Red-mauve, turns deep brown
Acetoacetic acid	Red or red-brown
Pyruvic acid	Deep gold yellow
α-Ketobutyric acid	Purple, fades to red-brown in 1–2 minutes
Salicylates	Stable purple
Phenothiazines	Purple
Phenol derivatives	Violet
p-Aminosalicylic acid	Red-brown
Antipyrines	Red
Acetophenetidines	Red
Cyanates	Red

Modified from Henry (1964)

CETYLTRIMETHYLAMMONIUM BROMIDE TEST

There are several inherited disorders which are associated with increased concentrations of the acid mucopolysaccharides in the tissues and in the urine. The acid mucopolysaccharides include the following: hyaluronic acid; chrondroitin sulfric acids A, B, and C; chrondroitin; keratosulfate; heparin; and heparin sulfuric acid. The mucopolysaccharides comprise much of the ground substance of connective tissue and disorders of mucopolysaccharide metabolism therefore include various defects of bone, cartilage, and connective tissue. Some of the disorders associated with excess urine mucopolysaccharides are Hurler's syndrome (gargoylism [autosomal recessive gene]), Hunter's syndrome (gargoylism [X-linked recessive gene]), Sanfilippo syndrome, Scheie's syndrome, Morquio's syndrome, and Maroteaux-Lamy syndrome.

The cetyltrimethylammonium bromide test (CTAB) is based on the reaction of the urinary mucopolysaccharides with quaternary ammonium salts to form a turbid solution and/or a precipitate. The urine must be tested at room temperature, because a cold urine will invariably give a false-positive test (Renuart 1966).

REAGENTS

1. Sodium citrate buffer, 1 M, ph 6.0—Dissolve 210 g of citric acid monohydrate in 800 ml of water. Slowly add 150 ml of 20 N sodium hydroxide. Mix well and allow to

cool to room temperature. Adjust the pH of the solution to 6.0 by the addition of 20 N sodium hydroxide. Dilute to a final volume of 1000 ml with distilled water.

2. 5% Cetyltrimethylammonium bromide reagent—Dissolve 50 g of cetyltrimethylammonium bromide (hexadecyltrimethylammonium bromide) in 1000 ml of the 1 M sodium citrate buffer. Both reagents are stable at room temperature (Buist 1968).

PROCEDURE

1. Place 1 ml of *clear* urine in a test tube and allow the urine to reach room temperature.
2. Add 6 drops of CTAB reagent and mix.
3. After 30 minutes observe for a cloudy or flocculent precipitate which indicates a positive test.

False-positive results occur if the urine is tested while cold, and also if there is a large number of cells present in the urine (Renuart 1966). False positives may also occur in very young children (Procopis et al. 1968).

Studies by Renuart (1966) using the CTAB test on urines from over 2000 patients with mental deficiency or other neurologic disorders showed that urines which contain chrondroitin sulfate B give a heavier precipitate with the CTAB test than those containing an equal concentration of heparitin sulfate.

DINITROPHENYLHYDRAZINE TEST

Several inborn errors of metabolism are associated with a markedly increased urinary excretion of keto-acids. The screening test utilizing the reagent 2,4-dinitrophenylhydrazine (DNPH) detects excessive amounts of a variety of keto compounds including α-keto acids as well as ketone bodies. Some inherited disorders which are associated with an excessive excretion of keto-acids are: phenylketonuria, maple-syrup urine disease, Lowe's syndrome, Oasthouse disease, and tyrosinosis.

Since ketone bodies also give a positive result with the DNPH test, care should be taken to compare the result with the ketone part of the R+M. It should be noted, however, that some α-keto acid disorders are also associated with the excretion of ketone bodies, i.e., maple-syrup urine disease (Thomas and Howell 1973). Also, there are some genetic disorders which are not associated with the excretion of α-keto acids but are associated with ketosis. Examples of these disorders are hyperglycinemia, isovaleric acidemia, and glycogen storage disease types 1, 3, 5, and 6 (Buist 1968).

REAGENTS

1. 2 N HCl—Add 16.7 ml of concentrated HCl to a 100 ml volumetric flask containing about 70 ml of distilled water.

Dilute to a total volume of 100 ml with distilled water and mix.

2. Dinitrophenylhydrazine reagent (0.1%)—Dissolve 100 mg of 2,4-dinitrophenylhydrazine in 100 ml of 2 N HCl. The reagent should be stored in a dark bottle in the refrigerator but must be brought to room temperature before testing (Buist 1968).

PROCEDURE
1. To 1 ml of *clear* urine in a test tube add 1 ml of DNPH reagent. Mix well.
2. Read the reaction at 10 minutes. A yellow or chalky white precipitate indicates a positive reaction.

If the mixture is allowed to sit for an hour or longer, a small red precipitate will form in the bottom of the tube as a result of normal amino acids in the urine. Renuart (1966) states that β-keto acids do not give a positive reaction with this procedure.

The DNPH test is usually moderately positive during the first days of life as a result of the normally increased excretion of pyruvic acid, acetoacetic acid, and β-ketoglutarate (Snyderman 1971).

CYANIDE—NITROPRUSSIDE TEST

The cyanide–nitroprusside test is widely used to detect urinary amino acids which contain a free sulfhydryl group or disulfide bond. A positive result therefore occurs in the presence of an excess amount of cystine, cysteine, homocystine, and homocysteine. In the reaction, the sodium cyanide solution reduces these compounds releasing free sulfhydryl groups from disulfide linkage, and the sodium nitroprusside reacts with the reduced free sulfhydryl group. The final color development is the net result of both the available reducible disulfides plus any preformed free sulfhydryl groups already present in the urine (Thomas and Howell 1973). Normally, the concentration of sulfhydryl in the urine is too low to give a color reaction.

REAGENTS
1. Concentrated ammonium hydroxide
2. 5% Sodium cyanide—Add 5 g of NaCN to distilled water and dilute to a total volume of 100 ml (POISONOUS!).
3. 5% Sodium nitroprusside—Add 5 g of sodium nitroprusside to distilled water and dilute to 100 ml. Both this and the previous reagent should be stored in a brown bottle in the refrigerator (Buist 1968). These reagents are best if made up fresh each time, but some labs make them up once a week (Smith 1977).

PROCEDURE
1. Place 1 ml of urine in a test tube and alkalinize to pH 6–8 using the NH₄OH.
2. Add 0.4 ml (12 drops) of the NaCN solution and mix well.
3. Allow to stand 10 minutes.
4. Add 1–3 drops of the sodium nitroprusside reagent, mix well, and observe for an immediate pink-red or magenta color which indicates a positive result.

A false-negative reaction will occur if the urine is too acidic (Buist 1968) or if the urine is too dilute (Smith 1977). It is very important to wait 10 minutes after the addition of the sodium cyanide to allow for complete freeing of sulfhydryl groups.

The cyanide–nitroprusside test will not detect cystathionine or methionine (Snyderman 1971, Buist 1968).

There is a variation of the cyanide–nitroprusside test which uses Acetest (Ames Co.) tablets. An Acetest tablet is placed in a spot depression plate, and a large drop of 10% sodium cyanide in 1 N NaOH is added to the tablet, followed quickly by a large drop of urine. The solution around the tablet is observed for a cherry-red color (Free and Free 1975).

NITROSONAPHTHOL TEST

There are several disorders which are associated with a marked alteration in the metabolism of tyrosine. These disorders include tyrosinosis, hereditary tyrosinemia with or without hepatorenal disease, transient tyrosinemia of the newborn, and severe liver dysfunction. The nitrosonaphthol test gives a positive result in the presence of tyrosine or its metabolites, including p-hydroxyphenylpyruvic acid, p-hydroxyphenyllactic acid, and p-hydroxyphenylacetic acid.

REAGENTS
1. 2.63 N Nitric acid—Add 1 part of concentrated nitric acid to 5 parts of distilled water.
2. Sodium nitrite solution—Dissolve 2.5 g of sodium nitrite in 100 ml of distilled water.
3. Nitrosonapthol reagent—Dissolve 100 mg of 1-nitroso-2-naphthol in 100 ml of 95% ethanol. The sodium nitrite and nitrosonaphthol solutions should be stored in the refrigerator (Perry et al. 1966).

PROCEDURE
1. Place 1 ml of the 2.63 N nitric acid in a test tube.
2. Add 1 drop of sodium nitrite.
3. Add 0.1 ml of nitrosonaphthol reagent and shake to mix.
4. Immediately add 3 drops of urine and mix well.
5. Observe for the presence of color for 5 minutes. The development of an orange to red color within 2–5 minutes

indicates a positive result, while the persistence of the original yellow color indicates a negative test.

NINHYDRIN TEST

The ninhydrin test detects the presence of excessive urinary amino acids and is positive in many different diseases involving aminoaciduria. It is especially useful for the detection of generalized aminoacidurias. However, the elevation of single amino acids may not be detected if the overall quantity of urinary amino acids is not increased. Positive results should be followed up by amino acid chromatography studies.

REAGENT

Ninhydrin solution—Dissolve 1 g of ninhydrin in 500 ml of 95% ethanol. Store in a brown bottle in the refrigerator (Buist 1968).

PROCEDURE

1. Place 1 ml of ninhydrin reagent in a test tube.
2. Add 3 drops of urine and mix.
3. Examine for color after 2 and 5 minutes. The presence of a blue or purple color, especially after 2 minutes, indicates that the urine may contain an excessive amount of one or more amino acids (Perry et al. 1966).

A very concentrated urine may give a false-positive result. Conversely, a very dilute urine may contain a significant amount of one amino acid and yet still give a negative result.

Perry et al. (1966) state that the ninhydrin test is not likely to detect the gross aminoaciduria found in Wilson's disease until the end of the first decade of life, at which time the symptoms of the disease may already be appearing. Therefore, a negative ninhydrin test on an infant's urine does not exclude Wilson's disease.

Porphyrins and Porphobilinogen

Porphyrins are complex iron-free cyclic substances which are intermediates in the biosynthetic pathway of heme (see Figure 5-3). They consist of four pyrrole rings linked by methene bridges to form a large ring structure (tetrapyrrole ring). The various types of porphyrins differ in the side chains which are present at the eight available positions on the pyrrole rings.

The main sites of porphyrin production are the bone marrow and the liver. Porphyrins formed in the bone marrow are intermediates in the synthesis of hemoglobin, whereas porphyrins formed in the liver and other tissues are intermediates for other heme proteins such as myoglobin.

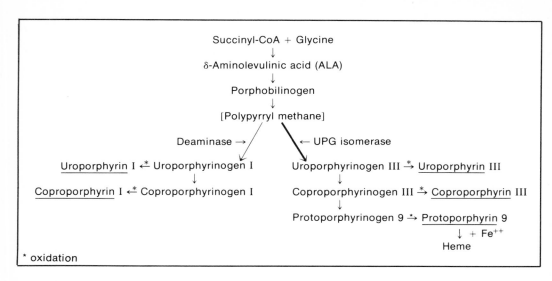

FIGURE 5-3   **Biosynthesis of heme.** (Porphyrins are *underlined*.)

TABLE 5-4					**Porphyrin and Porphyrin Precursors in the Urine**
Disorder	**Urinary Findings**				**Ref.**
	ALA	**PBG**	**CP**	**UR**	
Inherited					
Congenital erythropoietic porphyria (Gunther's disease)	N	N	↑ (I)	↑ ↑ (I)	
Acute intermittent porphyria (acute attack)	↑ ↑	↑ ↑	↑	N or ↑ *	
Variegate porphyria (chronic)	N	N	N or ↑	N or ↑	*
Variegate porphyria (acute)	↑ ↑	↑ ↑	↑	↑	*
Hereditary coproporphyria (acute)	N or ↑	N or ↑	↑ (III)	N	***
Acquired					
Lead intoxication	↑ ↑	N or sl ↑	↑ ↑ (III)	N or sl ↑ **	
Acquired porphyria cutanea tarda (Symptomatic porphyria)	N	N	↑	↑ ↑	

* Gray (1970)	N = Normal	ALA = δ-aminolevulinic acid
** Taddeni and Watson (1968)	sl ↑ = Slightly increased	PBG = porphobilinogen
*** Elder et al. (1972)	↑ = Increased	CP = coproporphyrins
	↑ ↑ = Greatly increased	UR = uroporphyrins
		$\frac{(I)}{(III)}$ = dominant type excreted

Overproduction of porphyrin intermediates and/or precursors by either the bone marrow or the liver causes increased urinary and fecal excretion of these substances as well as tissue accumulation. There are various disorders of porphyrin metabolism, some of which are inherited (e.g., congenital erythropoietic porphyria), and some of which are acquired (e.g., lead intoxication). Depending upon the disease, various porphyrins or precursors become elevated in the urine, blood, and/or feces. Table 5-4 lists some of the major porphyrias and the corresponding urinary findings.

Porphobilinogen and the porphyrinogens (uro-, copro-, and proto-) are colorless non-fluorescent substances, whereas the oxidized forms or the porphyrins are red pigments which exhibit fluorescence when viewed under ultraviolet light. Urine which contains large amounts of porphyrins may have a port-wine or burgundy color, or it may become dark red only after standing. The color of the urine depends on the type of porphyrin disorder.

The investigation of porphyrin disorders usually begins with screening tests for porphyrins or their precursors, ALA or porphobilinogen. The procedure for ALA (δ-aminolevulinic acid) will not be presented here, because this procedure is not a rapid screening test and also because it is usually performed in the chemistry laboratory. Positive screening procedures should be followed up by quantitation and fractionation studies.

Porphyrin Screening Test

In the porphyrin screening test, urinary porphyrins (coproporphyrin, uroporphyrin, and protoporphyrin) and extracted into acidified ethyl acetate and their fluorescence is viewed in ultraviolet light. Porphobilinogen, ALA, and the porphyrinogens are not detected by this method (Haining et al. 1969).

REAGENT
Glacial acetic acid/ethyl acetate—Mix 1 part glacial acetic acid with 4 parts of ethyl acetate.

PROCEDURE
1. Place 5 ml of urine in a glass centrifuge tube. (Do not use plastic tubes!) Add 3 ml of glacial acetic acid/ethyl acetate.
2. Cover tube and shake well. Allow the layers to separate or centrifuge to speed up separation.
3. Using a Wood's lamp, observe the upper layer for fluorescence and take a reading immediately. Blue fluorescence indicates negative or normal amounts of porphyrins. Violet to pink to red fluorescence indicates increasing levels of porphyrins. Results may be reported as normal, slightly elevated, moderately elevated, or grossly elevated, or they may be reported as normal through 4 +.

It is critical that a reading be taken as soon as the extracted specimen is placed in the ultraviolet light. On continued exposure to UV light, the porphyrin-containing layer will often develop an increased fluorescence, which can be misinterpreted as elevated porphyrins (Nutter and Labbé 1972).

The sensitivity of this test may be increased by performing the following modification after step #2 (Haining et al. 1969).

3. Transfer the upper layer into another glass tube and add 0.5 ml of 3 N HCl (25 ml concentrated HCl diluted to 100 ml with distilled water).
4. Shake well and observe under UV light. The porphyrins are extracted into the lower acid layer, while interfering substances remain in the organic phase. Acid greatly intensifies porphyrin fluorescence, and the fluorescence loses its bluish tint to become orange-red in color.

Watson-Schwartz Test

The Watson-Schwartz test detects porphobilinogen and urobilinogen and differentiates them by means of their solubility properties. The principle of the test is that porphobilinogen and urobilinogen react with Ehrlich's reagent to form red-colored aldehyde. Sodium acetate is added to increase the pH and to intensify color development. Extractions are performed to separate urobilinogen aldehyde from porphobilinogen aldehyde. Urobilinogen aldehyde is soluble in both chloroform and butanol. Porphobilinogen aldehyde is insoluble in both chloroform and butanol but is soluble in water.

The test should be performed on freshly voided urine which has been allowed to reach room temperature. When urine is allowed to stand before testing, the porphobilinogen may be oxidized to porphobilin which is not detected by this procedure. Also, if the urine is warm, a false-positive reaction may occur due to the "warm benzaldehyde reaction".

REAGENTS
1. Modified Ehrlich's reagent:
   p-dimethylaminobenzaldehyde—0.7 g
   concentrated HCl—150 ml
   distilled deionized H_2O—100 ml
   Mix and store in a brown bottle.
2. Saturated sodium acetate—Dissolve 1 kg of sodium acetate in 1 liter of water at 60°C.
3. Chloroform
4. Butanol

PROCEDURE
1. In a large test tube, combine 3 ml of urine and 3 ml of modified Ehrlich's reagent and mix.

2. Add 6 ml of saturated sodium acetate and mix well. A pink to red color indicates porphobilinogen, urobilinogen, or other Ehrlich-reacting substances (e.g., indole)

3. Add 3 ml of chloroform, shake well, and centrifuge briefly or allow the layers to settle out.

4. Porphobilinogen aldehyde is insoluble in chloroform and will remain in the aqueous or top layer, giving it a pink or red color. Urobilinogen aldehyde and other Ehrlich-reacting compounds are soluble in chloroform and so these colored compounds will be present in the chloroform (bottom) layer.

5. If both layers have a pink color, extract with chloroform again.

   Interpretation:
   Pink or red aqueous (top) layer = porphobilinogen
   Pink or red chloroform (bottom) layer = urobilinogen
      or other Ehrlich-reacting substances

If the top layer is pink or red, the following confirmatory step for porphobilinogen can be used.

6. Remove some of the supernatant or aqueous layer and add an equal amount of butanol. Mix well and allow to separate. The butanol layer will be on the top and the aqueous layer on the bottom. All known Ehrlich aldehyde compounds, except for porphobilinogen, will be extracted into the butanol layer. Porphobilinogen will remain in the aqueous (bottom) layer.

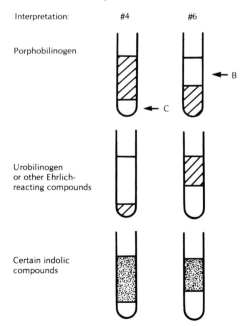

Interpretation: #4   #6

Porphobilinogen

                                               ← B

                                       ← C

Urobilinogen
or other Ehrlich-
reacting compounds

Certain indolic
compounds

(*Note:* The aldehyde derivatives of melanogen, serotonin, and some indoles are insoluble in chloroform but soluble in butanol [Bauer et al. 1968].)

It should be mentioned that there are some occasions in which both porphobilinogen and urobilinogen are present, but this is very rare.

Hoesch Test for Porphobilinogen

The Hoesch test uses Ehrlich's original reagent but is based on the inverse Ehrlich's reaction (i.e., of maintaining an acid solution by adding a small amount of urine to a relatively large volume of reagent) (Lamon et al. 1974). The procedure is specific for porphobilinogen; urobilinogen is not detected. As with all procedures for porphobilinogen, this test must be performed on fresh urine.

EHRLICH'S REAGENT
p-dimethylaminobenzaldehyde—20 g
HCl (6 mol/liter)—q.s. to 1000 ml
   First, make 1000 ml of 6 M HCl by mixing 500 ml of concentrated HCl and 500 ml of water. Then place 20 g of p-dimethylaminobenzaldehyde in a liter volumetric flask and q.s. to 1000 ml with the 6 M HCl. Reagent can be kept in a clear glass container for up to nine months (Lamon et al. 1974).

PROCEDURE
1. Place 2–3 ml of the Ehrlich's reagent in a test tube, and add 2 drops of fresh urine.
2. If porphobilinogen is present, a cherry-red color will instantly appear at the top of the solution and will spread throughout when the tube is agitated. Report as positive or negative for porphobilinogen.

The Hoesch test does not detect the low concentrations of porphobilinogen that are present in normal urine.

Bibliography

Abbott. Examination of urinary sediments: an atlas of use of Sternheimer Malbin staining technique. North Chicago, IL: Abbott Laboratories; 1961.

Alba's medical technology. 8th ed. Westlake, OR: Berkeley Scientific Publications; 1975.

Ames. Modern urine chemistry. Elkhart, IN: Ames Company, Division Miles Laboratories, Inc.; 1976.

Ames Company, Division Miles Laboratories, Inc. Ames Acetest reagent tablets. Elkhart, IN; 1975a; Package insert No. 2392AD. 2p.

Ames Company, Division Miles Laboratories, Inc. Ames Clinitest reagent tablets. Elkhart, IN; 1978a; Package insert No. 2920AD. 2p.

Ames Company, Division Miles Laboratories, Inc. C-Stix reagent strip. Elkhart, IN; 1975b; Package insert No. 7002AD. 2p.

Ames Company, Division Miles Laboratories, Inc. N-Multistix reagent strips for urinalysis. Elkhart, IN; 1979; Product profile No. 3157-799-50M. 4p.

Ames Company, Division Miles Laboratories, Inc. N-Multistix SG reagent strips. Elkhart, IN; 1981; Package insert No. 2592AD. 2p.

Ames Company, Division Miles Laboratories, Inc. Phenistix reagent strips for urinalysis. Elkhart, IN; 1978b; Package insert No. 2750AD. 2p.

Andrassy, K.; Ritz, E.; Koderisch, J.; Salzmann, W.; Bommer, J. Pseudoproteinuria in patients taking penicillin [letter]. Lancet 2(8081):154; 1978.

Arnow, L. E. Introduction to physiological and pathological chemistry. 7th ed. St. Louis: C.V. Mosby Co.; 1966.

Assa, S. Evaluation of urinalysis methods used in 35 Israeli laboratories. Clin. Chem. 23:126–128; 1977.

Bailey, R.R.; Dann, E.; Gilles, A.H.B.; Lynn, K.L.; Abernethy, M.H.; Neale, T.J. What the urine contains following athletic competition. N.Z. Med. J. 83:309–313; 1976.

Baker, F.J.; Silverton, R.E.; Luckcock, E.D. Introduction to medical laboratory technology. 4th ed. Washington: Butterworth & Co.; 1966.

Balant, L.P.; Fabre, J. Clinical significance of proteinuria. Compr. Ther. 4(10):54–62; 1978.

Bauer, J.D.; Ackerman, P.G.; Toro, G. Bray's clinical laboratory methods. 7th ed. St. Louis: C.V. Mosby Co.; 1968.

Beeler, M.F.; Henry, J.B. Melanogenuria: evaluation of several commonly used laboratory procedures. J. Am. Med. Assoc. 176:136–138; 1961.

Bennett, C.M.; Glassock, R.J. The dynamic kidney. Indianapolis: Eli Lilly and Co.; n.d.

Berman, L.B. When the urine is red. J. Am. Med. Assoc. 237:2753–2754; 1977.

Berman, L.B.; Schreiner, G.E.; Feys, J.O. Observations on the glitter-cell phenomenon. N. Engl. J. Med. 255:989–991; 1956.

Berry, H.K.; Leonard, C.; Peters, H.; Granger, M.; Chunekamrai, N. Detection of metabolic disorders: chromatographic procedures and interpretation of results. Clin. Chem. 14:1033–1065; 1968.

Bio-Dynamics/bmc, Division of Boehringer Mannheim. Chemstrip 8 dip and read test. Indianapolis; 1979a; Package insert No. 369551. 2p.

Bio-Dynamics/bmc, Division of Boehringer Mannheim. Chemstrip L dip and read test for leukocytes in urine. Indianapolis; 1979b; Package insert No. 398608. 1p.

BMC. Urinalysis with Chemstrip. Indianapolis: Bio-Dynamics/bmc, Division of Boehringer Mannheim; 1978.

Boggs, D.R.; Winkelstein, A. White cell manual. 3rd ed. Philadelphia: F.A. Davis Co.; 1975.

Bowie, L.; Smith, S.; Gochman, N. Characteristics of binding between reagent-strip indicators and urinary proteins. Clin. Chem. 23:128–130; 1977.

Boyd, P.J.R. Haematuria. Br. Med. J. 2(6084):445–446; 1977.

Bradley, G.M. Urinary screening tests in the infant and young child. Med. Clin. North Am. 55:1457–1471; 1971.

Bradley, M.; Schumann, G.B.; Ward, P.C.J. Examination of urine. Henry, J.B., ed. Todd-Sanford-Davidson's clinical diagnosis and management by laboratory methods. 16th ed. Philadelphia: W.B. Saunders Co.; 1979: 559–634.

Brandt, R.: Guyer, K. E.; Banks, W.L., Jr. Urinary glucose and vitamin C. Am. J. Clin. Pathol. 68:592–594; 1977.

Bright, T.C.; White, K.; Peters, P.C. Significance of hematuria after trauma. J. Urol. 120:455–456; 1978.

Brody, L.H.; Salladay, J.R.; Armbruster, K. Urinalysis and the urinary sediment. Med. Clin. North Am. 55:243–266; 1971.

Buist, N.R.M. Set of simple side-room urine tests for detection of inborn errors of metabolism. Br. Med. J. 2:745–749; 1968.

Burton, J.R.; Rowe, J.W. Quantitation of casts in urine sediment. Ann. Intern. Med. 83:518–519; 1975.

Cannon, D.C. The identification and pathogenesis of urine casts. Lab. Med. 10:8–11; 1979.

Chudwin, D.S.; Chesney, P.J.; Mischler, E.H.; Chesney, R.W. Hematuria associated with carbenicillin and other semisynthetic penicillins. Am. J. Dis. Child. 133:98–99; 1979.

Clemens, A.H.; Hurtle, R.L. Automatic system for urine analysis: I. System design and development; II. Evaluation of the system. Clin. Chem. 18:789–799; 1972.

Cloonan, M.J.; Donald, T.G.; Neale, C.; Wilcken, D.E.L. The detection of myoglobin in urine and its application to the diagnosis of myocardial infarction. Pathology 8:313–320; 1976.

Court, J.M.; Davies, H.E.; Ferguson, R. Diastix and ketodiastix: a new semiquantitative test for glucose in urine. Med. J. Aust. 1:525–528; 1972.

Crook, W.G. Food allergy and albuminuria [letter]. J. Pediatr. 90:857–858; 1977.

D'Eramo, E.M.; McAnear, J.T. The significance of urinalysis in treatment of hospitalized dental patients. Oral Surg. 38:36–41; 1974.

de Wardener, H.E. The kidney. 3rd ed. Boston: Little, Brown and Co.; 1967.

Diggs, L.W. Erythrocyte disorders and responses. Miller, S.E.; Weller, J.M., eds. Textbook of clinical pathology. 8th ed. Baltimore: Williams & Wilkins Co.; 1971: 82–119.

DiSalvo, A.F.; Scarborough, L.L. Screening for phenylketonuria (PKU) in South Carolina. J. S.C. Med. Assoc. 74:529–531; 1978.

Douglas, A.P.; Kerr, D.N.S. A short textbook of kidney diseases. Great Britain: Pitman Press; 1971.

Eastham, R.D. A laboratory guide to clinical diagnosis. Great Britain: John Wright & Sons Ltd.; 1976.

Efron, M.L. Aminoaciduria. N. Engl. J. Med. 272:1058–1067; 1965.

Efron, M.L.; Young, D.; Moser, H.W.; MacCready, R.A. A simple chromatographic screening test for the detection of disorders of amino acid metabolism: a technic using whole blood or urine collected on filter paper. N. Engl. J. Med. 270:1378–1383; 1964.

Elder, G.H.; Gray, C.H.; Nicholson, D.C. The porphyrias: a review. J. Clin. Pathol. 25:1013–1033; 1972.

Erslev, A.J.; Gabuzda, T.G. Pathophysiology of blood. Philadelphia: W.B. Saunders Co.; 1975.

Exton, W.G. A simple and rapid quantitative test for albumin in urine. J. Lab. Clin. Med. 10:722–734; 1925.

Frankel, S. Chemical examination. Frankel, S.; Reitman, S., eds. Gradwohl's clinical laboratory methods and diagnosis. 6th ed. St. Louis: C.V. Mosby Co.; 1963a: 1808–1836.

Frankel, S. Microscopic examination. Frankel, S.; Reitman, S., eds. Gradwohl's clinical laboratory methods and diagnosis. 6th ed. St. Louis: C.V. Mosby Co.; 1963b: 1845–1865.

Fred, H.L. More on grossly bloody urine of runners [editorial]. Arch. Intern. Med. 138:1610–1611; 1978.

Fred, H.L.; Natelson, E.A. Grossly bloody urine of runners. South Med. J. 70:1394–1396; 1977.

Free, A.H.; Free, H.M. Rapid convenience urine tests: their use and misuse. Lab. Med. 9(12):9–17; 1978.

Free, A.H.; Free, H.M. Urinalysis in clinical laboratory practice. Cleveland: CRC Press, Inc.; 1975.

Free, A.H.; Free, H.M. Urodynamics: concepts relating to urinalysis. Elkhart, IN: Ames Company, Division Miles Laboratories, Inc.; 1974.

Freni, S.C.; Dalderup, L.M.; Oudegeest, J.J.; Wensveen, N. Erythrocyturia, smoking, and occupation. J. Clin. Pathol. 30:341–344; 1977.

Frimpter, G.W. Aminoacidurias due to inherited disorders of metabolism. N. Engl. J. Med. 289:835–841, 895–901; 1973.

Gambino, R., ed. The routine urine microscopic—eliminated by a new test strip. G/R Publications, Inc.; Lab Report for Physicians 3(19):39–40; 1981.

Gatenby, P.A.; Shagrin, J.M.; Tiller, D.J. The use of Microstix in the diagnosis of urinary tract infections. Med. J. Aust. 2:675–677; 1974.

Goldberg, H.E. Principles of refractometry. Buffalo, NY: American Optical Co.; 1965.

Gray, C.H. Porphyrias. Thompson, R.H.S.; Wootton, I.D.P., eds. Biochemical disorders in human disease. 3rd ed. London: Churchill Livingstone Publishers; 1970.

Greenhill, A.; Gruskin, A.B. Laboratory evaluation of renal function. Pediatr. Clin. North Am. 23:661–679; 1976.

Guthrie, R.; Susi, A. A simple phenylalanine method for detecting phenylketonuria in large populations of newborn infants. Pediatrics 32:338–343; 1963.

Haber, M.H. Interference contrast microscopy for identification of urinary sediments. Am. J. Clin. Pathol. 57:316–319; 1972.

Haber, M.H. Urine casts: their microscopy and clinical significance. 2nd ed. Chicago: American Society of Clinical Pathologists; 1976.

Haber, M.H.; Lindner, L.E. Surface ultrastructure of urinary casts. Am. J. Clin. Pathol. 68:547–552; 1977.

Haber, M.H.; Lindner, L.E.; Ciofalo, L.N. Urinary casts after stress. Lab. Med. 10:351–355; 1979.

Hager, C.B.; Free, A.H. Urine urobilinogen as a component of routine urinalysis. Am. J. Med. Technol. 36:227–233; 1970.

Haining, R.G.; Hulse, T.; Labbé, R.F. Rapid porphyrin screening of urine, stool, and blood. Clin. Chem. 15:460–466; 1969.

Hansen, O.H.; Hansen, A.; Vibild, O. The relationship of lipuria to the fat embolism syndrome. Acta Chir. Scand. 139:421–424; 1973.

Henry, J.B. Clinical chemistry. Davidson, I.; Henry, J.B., eds. Todd-Sanford's clinical diagnosis by laboratory methods. 15th ed. Philadelphia: W.B. Saunders Co.; 1974; 516–664.

Henry, R.J. Clinical chemistry principles and technics. New York: Hoeber Medical Division, Harper & Row; 1964.

Hepler, O.E. Manual of clinical laboratory methods. 4th ed. Springfield, IL: Charles C Thomas; 1949.

Hillman, R.S.; Finch, C.A. Red cell manual. 4th ed. Philadelphia: F.A. Davis Co.; 1974.

Hinberg, I.H.; Katz, L.; Waddell, L. Sensitivity of in vitro diagnostic dipstick tests to urinary protein. Clin. Biochem. 11(2):62–64; 1978.

Hoffman, W.S. The biochemistry of clinical medicine. 4th ed. Chicago: Year Book Medical Publishers, Inc.; 1970.

Howanitz, P.J.; Howanitz, J.H. Carbohydrates. Henry, J.B., ed. Todd-Sanford-Davidson's clinical diagnosis and management by laboratory methods. 16th ed. Philadelphia: W.B. Saunders Co.; 1979: 153–188.

James, G.P.; Bee, D.E.; Fuller, J.B. Accuracy and precision of urinary pH determinations using two commercially available dipsticks. Am. J. Clin. Pathol. 70:368–374; 1978a.

James, G.P.; Bee, D.E.; Fuller, J.B. Proteinuria: accuracy and precision of laboratory diagnosis by dip-stick analysis. Clin. Chem. 24:1934–1939; 1978b.

James, G.P.; Paul, K.L.; Fuller, J.B. Urinary nitrite and urinary-tract infection. Am. J. Clin. Pathol. 70:671–678; 1978c.

James, J.A. Proteinuria and hematuria in children: diagnosis and assessment. Pediatr. Clin. North Am. 23:807–816; 1976.

Juel, R.; Steinrauf, M.A. Refractometry. Hicks, R.; Schenken, J.R.; Steinrauf, M.A., eds. Laboratory instrumentation. San Francisco: Harper & Row; 1974: 99–111.

Kachmar, J.F. Proteins and amino acids. Tietz, N.W., ed. Fundamentals of clinical chemistry. Philadelphia: W.B. Saunders Co.; 1970: 177–262.

Kishel, M.; Lichty, P. Some diaper brands give false-positive test for PKU [letter]. N. Engl. J. Med. 300:200; 1979.

Kissner, P.Z. Proteinuria and the nephrotic syndrome. Weller, J.M., ed. Fundamentals of nephrology. San Francisco: Harper & Row; 1979: 226–234.

Krupp, M.A.; Sweet, N.J.; Jawetz, E.; Biglieri, E.G.; Roe, R.L.; Camargo, C.A. Physician's handbook. 19th ed. Los Altos, CA: Lange Medical Publications; 1979.

Kurtzman, N.A.; Rogers, P.W. A handbook of urinalysis and urinary sediment. Springfield, IL: Charles C Thomas; 1974.

Kusumi, R.K.; Grover, P.J.; Kunin, C.M. Rapid detection of pyuria by leukocyte esterase activity. J. Am. Med. Assoc. 245:1653–1655; 1981.

Lamon, J.; With, T.K.; Redeker, A.G. The Hoesch test: bedside screening test for urinary porphobilinogen in patients with suspected porphyria. Clin. Chem. 20:1438–1440; 1974.

Latner, A.L. Cantarow and Trumper's clinical biochemistry. 7th ed. Philadelphia: W.B. Saunders Co.; 1975.

Lee, R. All that is green is not PKU [letter]. Pediatrics 62:859; 1978.

Levinson, S.A.; MacFate, R.P. Clinical laboratory diagnosis. 7th ed. Philadelphia: Lea & Febiger; 1969.

Lippman, R.W. Urine and the urinary sediment. 2nd ed. Springfield, IL: Charles C Thomas; 1957.

Lytton, B. Bleeding from the urinary tract. Med. Times 105(10):27–35; 1977.

Markowitz, H.; Wobig, G.H. Quantitative method for estimating myoglobin in urine. Clin. Chem. 23:1689–1693; 1977.

Mayes, P.A. Ketone bodies. Brownsville, TX: Proficiency Testing Service, American Association of Bioanalysts; 1973; Test of the Month No. 16. 4p.

McNeely, M.D.D. Urinalysis. Sonnenwirth, A.C.; Jarett, L., eds. Gradwohl's clinical laboratory methods and diagnosis. 8th ed. St. Louis: C.V. Mosby Co.; 1980: 478–503.

McQueen, E.G.; Sydney, M.B. Composition of urinary casts. Lancet 1:397–398; 1966.

Meyers, F.H.; Jawetz, E.; Goldfien, A. Review of medical pharmacology. 6th ed. Los Altos, CA: Lange Medical Publications; 1978.

Miale, J.B. Laboratory medicine: hematology. 5th ed. St. Louis: C.V. Mosby Co.; 1977.

Monte-Verde, D.; Nosanchuk, J.S.; Rudy, M.A.; Ziemba, R.; Anuskiewcz, K. Unknown crystals in the urine. Lab. Med. 10:299–302; 1979.

Murphy, J.E.; Henry, J.B. Evaluation of renal function, and water, electrolyte, and acid-base balance. Henry, J.B.; Statland, B.E., eds. Todd-Sanford-Davidson's clinical diagnosis and management by laboratory methods. 16th ed. Philadelphia: W.B. Saunders Co.; 1979: 135–152.

Muth, R.G. Renal medicine. Springfield, IL: Charles C Thomas; 1978.

Nahata, M.C.; McLeod, D.C. Noneffect of oral urinary copper ascorbic acid on reduction glucose test. Diabetes Care 1(1):34–35; 1978.

Nutter, J.; Labbé, R.F. Improved screening tests for porphyrin. Clin. Chem. 18:739; 1972.

Ottaviano, P.J.; DiSalvo, A.F. Quality control in the clinical laboratory: a procedural text. Baltimore: University Park Press; 1977.

Papper, S. Clinical nephrology. 2nd ed. Boston: Little, Brown and Company; 1978.

Peele, J.D., Jr.; Gadsden, R.H.; Crews, R. Evaluation of Ames' "Clini-Tek". Clin. Chem. 23:2238–2241; 1977a.

Peele, J.D., Jr.; Gadsden, R.H.; Crews, R. Semi-automated vs. visual reading of urinalysis dipsticks. Clin. Chem. 23:2242–2246; 1977b.

Perry, T.L.; Hansen, S.; MacDougall, L. Urinary screening tests in the prevention of mental deficiency. J. Can. Med. Assoc. 95:89–95; 1966.

Pitts, R.F. Physiology of the kidney and body fluids. 2nd ed. Chicago: Year Book Medical Publishers, Inc.; 1968.

Procopis, P.G.; Turner, B.; Ruxton, J.T.; Brown, D.A. Screening tests for mucopolysaccharidosis. J. Ment. Defic. Res. 12:13–17; 1968.

Pruzanski, W. Proteinuria: laboratory tests, diagnostic and prognostic significance. Brownsville, TX: Proficiency Testing Service, American Association of Bioanalysts; 1975; Test of the Month No. 27. 4p.

Pryor, J.S. Proteinuria. Br. Med. J. 2(6082):307–308; 1977.

Race, G.J.; White, M.G. Basic urinalysis. San Francisco: Harper & Row; 1979.

Randolph, M.F.; Morris, K. Instant screening for bacteriuria in children: analysis of a dipstick. J. Pediatr. 84:246–248; 1974.

Rasoulpour, M.; McLeon, R.H.; Raye, J.; Shah, B.L. Pseudohematuria in neonates. J. Pediatr. 92:852–853; 1978.

Ravel, R. Clinical laboratory medicine. 3rd ed. Chicago: Year Book Medical Publishers, Inc.; 1978.

Renuart, A.W. Screening for inborn errors of metabolism associated with mental deficiency or neurologic disorders or both. N. Engl. J. Med. 274:384–387; 1966.

Rényi-Vámos, F.; Babics, A. Anuria: therapeutic experiences. New York: Pitman Publishing Corp.; 1972. Translated from the Hungarian by A. Deak.

Ritchie, R.F. Specific proteins. Henry, J.B., ed. Todd-Sanford-Davidson's clinical diagnosis and management by laboratory methods. 16th ed. Philadelphia: W.B. Saunders Co.; 1979: 228–258.

ROCOM. Urine under the microscope. Nutley, NJ: ROCOM, Division of Hoffman-LaRoche Inc.; 1975.

Rutecki, G.J.; Goldsmith, C.; Schreiner, G.E. Characterization of protein in urinary casts. N. Engl. J. Med. 284:1049–1052; 1971.

Schreiner, G.E. The identification and clinical significance of casts. Arch. Intern. Med. 99:356–369; 1957.

Schreiner, G.E. The nephrotic syndrome. Strauss, M.B.; Welt, L.G., eds. Diseases of the kidney. Boston: Little, Brown and Co.; 1963: 503–636.

Schreiner, G.E. Urinary sediments. New York: Medcom, Inc.; 1969. (Famous teachings in modern medicine).

Scriver, C.R. Screening newborns for hereditary metabolic disease. Pediatr. Clin. North Am. 12:807–821; 1965.

Shaw, S.T., Jr.; Benson, E.S. Renal function and its evaluation. Davidson, I.; Henry, J.B., eds. Todd-Sanford's clinical diagnosis by laboratory methods. 15th ed. Philadelphia: W.B. Saunders Co.; 1974: 84–98.

Simmons, J.S.; Gentskow, C.J. Medical and public health laboratory methods. Philadelphia: Lea & Febiger; 1955.

Sisson, J.A. Handbook of clinical pathology. Philadelphia: J.B. Lippincott Co.; 1976.

Smith, A. Evaluation of the nitroprusside test for the diagnosis of cystinuria. Med. J. Aust. 2(5):153–155; 1977.

Smith, B.C.; Peake, M.J.; Fraser, C.G. Urinalysis by use of multi-test reagent strips: two dipsticks compared. Clin. Chem. 23:2337–2340; 1977.

Smith, D.; Young, W.W. Effect of large-dose ascorbic acid on the two-drop Clinitest determination. Am. J. Hosp. Pharm. 34:1347–1349; 1977.

Snyderman, S.E. Diagnosis of metabolic disease. Pediatr. Clin. North Am. 18:199–208; 1971.

Sobotka, H.; Luisada-Opper, A.V.; Reiner, M. A new test for bilirubin in urine. Am. J. Clin. Pathol. 23:607–609; 1953.

Sotelo-Avila, C.; Gooch, W.M., III. Clinical usefulness of serum and urine osmolality. J. Tenn. Med. Assoc. 69(2):110–113; 1976.

Stedman's medical dictionary. 23rd ed. Baltimore: Williams & Wilkins Co.; 1976.

Sternheimer, R. A supravital cytodiagnostic stain for urinary sediments. J. Am. Med. Assoc. 231:8; 1975.

Sternheimer, R.; Malbin, B. Clinical recognition of pyelonephritis, with a new stain for urinary sediments. Am. J. Med. 11:312; 1951.

Stryer, L. Biochemistry. San Francisco: W.H. Freeman and Co.; 1975.

Stuber, A. Screening tests and chromatography for the detection of inborn errors of metabolism. Clin. Chim. Acta 36:309–313; 1972.

Sweeney, M.J.; Forland, M. Methods of diagnosing renal disease: urinalysis. Stein, J.H., ed. Nephrology. San Francisco: Grune & Stratton; 1980: 64–78. (Dietschy, J.M., ed. The science and practice of clinical medicine; vol. 7).

Taddeini, L.; Watson, C.J. The clinical porphyrias. Semin. Hematol. 5:335–369; 1968.

Thomas, G.H.; Howell, R.R. Selected screening tests for genetic metabolic diseases. Chicago: Year Book Medical Publishers, Inc.; 1973.

Thompson, D.M. Hematuria associated with soda pop drinking [letter]. J. Am. Med. Assoc. 239:193; 1978.

Tietz, N.W., ed. Fundamentals of clinical chemistry. Philadelphia: W.B. Saunders Co.; 1976.

Triger, D.R.; Smith, J.W.G. Survival of urinary leucocytes. J. Clin. Pathol. 19:443–447; 1966.

Vidler, J.; Wilcken, B. Prevalence of unsuspected urinary bacterial contamination: effects of screening tests for detection of inborn errors of metabolism. Clin. Chim. Acta 82:173–178; 1978.

Wagoner, R.D.; Holley, K.E. Parenchymal renal disease: clinical and pathologic features. Knox, F.G., ed. Textbook of renal pathophysiology. San Francisco: Harper & Row; 1978: 226–253.

Waife, S.O., ed. Diabetes mellitus. 8th ed. Indianapolis: Eli Lilly and Co.; 1979.

Weisberg, H.F. Water, electrolytes, acid-base, and oxygen. Davidson, I.; Henry, J.B., eds. Todd-Sanford's clinical diagnosis by laboratory methods. 15th ed. Philadelphia: W.B. Saunders Co.; 1974: 772–803.

Weller, J.M. Examination of the urine. Weller, J.M., ed. Fundamentals of nephrology. San Francisco: Harper & Row; 1979: 79–86.

Weller, J.M. The urinary system. Miller, S.E.; Weller, J.M., eds. Textbook of clinical pathology. 8th ed. Baltimore: Williams & Wilkins Co.; 1971: 528–555.

White, W.L.; Frankel, S., eds. Seiverd's chemistry for medical technologists. 2nd ed. St. Louis: C.V. Mosby Co.; 1965.

Wilson, D.M. Urinalysis and other tests of renal function. Minn. Med. 58:9–17; 1975.

Wirth, W.A.; Thompson, R.L. The effect of various conditions and substances on the results of laboratory procedures. Am. J. Clin. Pathol. 43:579–590; 1965.

Wolf, A.V. Urinary concentrative properties. Am. J. Med. 32:329–332; 1962.

Wright, W.T. Cell counts in urine. Arch. Intern. Med. 103:76–78; 1959.

Zimmer, J.G.; Dewey, R.; Waterhouse, C.; Terry, R. The origin and nature of anisotropic urinary lipids in the nephrotic syndrome. Ann. Intern. Med. 54:205–214; 1961.

Zimmerman, H.J. Evaluation of the function and integrity of the liver. Henry, J.B., ed. Todd-Sanford-Davidson's clinical diagnosis and management by laboratory methods. 16th ed. Philadelphia: W.B. Saunders Co.; 1979: 305–346.

Index

Page numbers in *italics* refer to figures. If a figure and its legend are on different pages, the page number in italics refers to the page on which the legend is found. Numerals followed by a "t" indicate a table.

Acetest tablets, 46, 258
Acetic acid 2%, 75, *79*, *137*
Acetoacetic acid, 43–45
Acetone, 43–45
Acid urine crystals, 83–100, *85–86*
Acidosis, 24–25
Afferent arteriole, 3
Air bubbles, 125, *128*, *237*
Albumin, dipstick procedure and, 30
Aldosterone, 6
Alkali test, 246
Alkaline tide, 25
Alkaline urine crystals, 101–107, *101*
Alkalosis, 25
Alkaptonuria, 245
    urine color in, 12
Allograft rejection, 111
Aminoaciduria, 251–252
    generalized, 259
    no-threshold, 251
    overflow, 251
    renal-transport, 251
    secondary, 251–252
δ-Aminolevulinic acid, 261, *260*
Ammonium biurate crystals, 84t, 105–107, *101*, *107*, *179*, *181*, *183*
    spheroid, *107*, *183*, *185*
Ammonium sulfate test, 55
Ampicillin crystals, 98
Anthocyanins, 12
Antidiuretic hormone, 6
Anuria, 6
Artifacts, 122–128

Ascorbic acid, 242–243. *See also* Vitamin C
Azure A, 11t, 12

Bacteria, 116–117, *116*, *137*, *185*, *201*, *209*, *217*
Bacterial cast, *213*
Bacteriuria, 64–65
Bence-Jones protein, 33–35
    heat precipitation test for, 35
    multiple myeloma and, 34
    toluene sulfonic acid test for, 35
Benedict's qualitative test, 42–43
Bile. *See* Bilirubin
Bilirubin, 55–63
    foam test for, 60–61
    Harrison spot test for, 61
    Ictotest for, 60
    normal pathway of, *56*
    reagent test-strips for, 59–60
    screening tests for, 59–61
    Smith iodine test for, 61
Bilirubin crystals, 84t, 98, *100*, *169*, *171*
Bilirubin diglucuronide, 55
Bilirubin stain, *139*, *169*, *171*, *197*, *199*, *207*, *213*
Bilirubinuria, 13, 55–61
Biliverdin, 12, 59
Bladder catheterization, 7
Blood, occult, 48–55
    hematest for, 54–55
    reagent test-strips for, 53–54
    screening tests for, 52–55

Bowman's capsule, 4
Bowman's space, 4
Bromine test, 246–247
Bromthymol blue, 18, 26

Calcium carbonate crystals, 84t, 103, *101, 105*
Calcium oxalate crystals, 84t, 89–90, *85, 89–90, 141, 149, 151, 153, 155, 235*
Calcium phosphate crystals, 84t, 103–105, *101, 105, 177, 179, 205*
Calcium phosphate plates, *101, 105, 177, 179, 205*
Calcium sulfate crystals, 84t, 92, *86*
Calculi (stones), 83
Candida albicans, 117
Carbonic anhydrase, 5
Casts, 107–116, *109–115, 185–215*
  bent, *185*
  bilirubin-stained, *197, 199, 207, 213*
  broad, 107–108, *201, 215*
  classification of, 108
  cylindroids vs, 117–118
  epithelial cell, 111, *113, 211*
  fatty, 115–116, *115*
  formation of, 107
  granular, 111, *113, 199–207*
  hyaline, 108, *109, 185–191*
  mixed, *197, 211, 213, 215*
  red cell, 108–109, *111, 191, 193, 215*
  reporting number of, 72–73
  size and shape of, 107–108
  waxy, 111–115, *115, 207–211*
  white cell, 109–111, *111, 145, 189, 195–199*
Catheterization, bladder, 7
Cells, 74–81
  epithelial, 79–81, *80–82*
  erythrocytes, 74–77, *75–76*
  leukocytes, 77–79, *77–79*
Centrifugation, 72
Cetyltrimethylammonium bromide test, 253t, 255–256
Chemical examination, 21–67
Chemstrip L, 243–244
Chemstrip 8, 22
Chemstrip 9, 243–244
Children and specimen collection, 8
Chloroform, 9
Cholesterol, 120
Cholesterol crystals, 84t, 96–97, *86, 96*
Chyluria, 96–97
Cirrhosis, 56, 94

Clean-catch specimen, 7–8
Clean-voided midstream specimen, 7–8
Clini-Tek, 66
Clinilab, 67
Clinitest, 40–42
Cloth fibers, 124–125, *124–125, 227–235*
Copper reduction test, 40–43
Countercurrent multiplication, 5
Crystals, 83–107, 84t, *85–86, 101*
  acid urine, 83–100, *85–86*
  alkaline urine, 101–107, *101*
  ammonium biurate, 105–107, *107, 179–185*
  amorphous phosphate, 102–103, *103, 171, 173, 177, 179, 205, 237*
  amorphous urate, 90, *91, 143, 153, 155, 193, 207, 221, 225, 235*
  calcium carbonate, 103, *105*
  calcium oxalate, 89–90, *89–90, 141, 149–155, 235*
  calcium phosphate, 103–105, *105, 177, 179, 205*
  calcium sulfate, 92, *86*
  cholesterol, 96–97, *96*
  cystine, 92–94, *93, 157–163*
  drug, 97–98, *97–100*
  hippuric acid, 90, *91, 155*
  leucine, 94, *94*
  radiographic dye, 98, *98–100, 167–169*
  reporting number of, 74
  sodium urate, 90–92, *92, 155–157*
  solubility characteristics of, 83, 84t
  starch, 122, *123, 225, 227*
  triple phosphate, 102, *102, 171–177*
  tyrosine, 94–96, *95, 165–167*
  uric acid, 83, *86–88, 143–151*
C-Stix, 242
Cushing's syndrome, 37
Cyanide–nitroprusside test, 92, 253t, 257–258
Cylindroids, 117–118, *118, 215*
Cysteine, 257
Cystine, 257
Cystine crystals, 84t, 92–94, *86, 93, 157–163*
  clustered, *161*
  layered or laminated, *159*
  pitted surface of, *163*
  pseudocast formation of, *163*
  thick, *161*
  unequal sides of, *159*
  various sizes of, *163*
Cystitis, 7

Debris, *153*
Diabetes insipidus, 14
Diabetes mellitus
   ketoacidosis in, 44–45
   specific gravity in, 14
   symptoms of, 36
Diacetic acid, 43–45
Diaper fibers, 124, *125, 227, 231*
p-dimethylaminobenzaldehyde, 62, 63, 262,
   264
Dinitrophenylhydrazine test, 253t, 256–257
Drug crystals, 97–98, *97–100*

Efferent arteriole, 4
Ehrlich's qualitative test, 63
Ehrlich's reaction, 62
Ehrlich's reagent, 63, 262, 264
Enterobius vermicularis, 129, 131, 237, 239
Eosin stain, 70
Epithelial cells, 79–81, *80–82, 135, 189, 197,
     209, 219, 221*
   bilirubin-stained, *139*
   renal tubular, 80, *80, 135, 139*
   reporting number of, 74
   squamous, 81, *82, 135, 141, 153, 161, 163,
     183, 195, 237*
   transitional, 81, *81, 82, 135, 141*
Epithelial cell cast, 111, *113, 211*
Erythrocytes, 74–77, *75–76.* See also Red
   blood cells
Exercise and hematuria, 50
Exton's reagent, 31

Fat bodies
   doubly refractive, 120
   oval, 120, *120–122, 221–225*
Fat droplets, 120, *120–122, 171, 221*
Fatty casts, 115–116, *115*
Fecal contaminants, 125, *129*
Ferric chloride test
   homogentisic acid, 245
   inborn errors of metabolism, 253t, 254,
     255t
   melanin, 246
   phenylketonuria and, 250
   reactants in, 253t, 255t
Ferritin, 51

Fibers, 124–125, *124–126*
   bilirubin-stained, 197
   dark edged, *229*
   diaper, 124, *125, 227, 231*
   indentations in, *233*
   nodular indentations on, 125, *126, 233,
     235*
   striated, *233*
   thick nodular border of, *235*
   thick rolled edged, *231*
   waxy cast vs, *231*
Film test, 246
Focus, microscopic, 72, *73*
Formaldehyde, 9
Formalin, 8–9
Fouchet's reagent, 61
Fructose, 37

Galactose, 37
Galactosemia, 253t, 254
Gerhardt's test, 47–48
Ghost cells, 49, 74, *75*
Glass fragments, 125, *127*
Glitter cells, 78
Glomerular disease, 108
Glomerulonephritis, 7, 27–28, 49
Glomerulus, 2–4, *4*
Gluconeogenesis, 36
Glucose, 36–43
   glucose oxidase test for, 38–40
   normal renal threshold for, 5, 36
   reagent strips for, 38t
Glucose oxidase test, 38–40
Glucuronic acid, 55
Glycogenolysis, 36
Glycosuria, 36–38
   alimentary, 36
   renal, 37
   timed specimens in, 9
Granular casts, 111, *113, 145, 169, 207, 215,
     221*
   bilirubin-stained, *169, 197, 199, 207, 213,
     215*
   broad, *201, 215*
   coarse, *113, 203, 205*
   fine, *113, 145, 199, 201, 203, 209, 219, 229*
Granular cylindroid, *215*
Granular inclusions, *191*
Guthrie test, 248–249

Hair, 125, *127*
Ham test, 243
Haptoglobin, 50–51
Harrison spot test, 61
Hart's test, 48
Heat and acetic acid test, 32
Heller's ring test, 32–33
Hematest, 54–55
Hematuria, 12, 49–50, 76
Heme biosynthesis, *260*
Hemoglobinuria, 12, 50–52
  ammonium sulfate test for, 55
Hemosiderin, 51, 243
  Ham test for, 243
  Prussian blue reaction for, 243
  Rous test for, 243
Hepatitis, viral, 56, 94
Hippuric acid crystals, 84t, 90, *86, 91, 155*
Hoesch test, 264
Homocysteine, 257
Homocystine, 257
Homogentisic acid, 12, 245–246
  alkali test for, 246
  ferric chloride test for, 245
  film test for, 246
Hunter's syndrome, 255
Hurler's syndrome, 253t, 255
Hyaline casts, 108, *109, 185, 189*
  bent, *187*
  granular inclusions and, *191*
Hyaline cylindroid, 72, *73, 215*
β-Hydroxybutyric acid, 43–48
p-Hydroxyphenylacetic acid, 258
p-Hydroxyphenyllactic acid, 258
p-Hydroxyphenylpyruvic acid, 249t, 255t,
  258, *245*
Hypaque crystals, 98, *98, 99*
Hyperglycemia, 36–37
Hypersthenuria, 14
Hyposthenuria, 14
Hypotonic urine, 78, *77, 135*

Ictotest, 60
Indole, 62, 63
Infant specimen collection, 8
Instrumentation, 65–67
  Clinilab, 67
  Clini-Tek, 66
  Urotron, 66–67

Iodine stain, 70
Isosthenuria, 14

Jaundice, 56–59
  hemolytic, 58–59, *58*
  hepatic, 56–57, *57*
  obstructive, 57–58, *58*
    urine color in, 12

Ketoacidosis, 44–45
Keto-acids, increased, 256
Ketones, 43–48
  Acetest tablets for, 46
  acetoacetic acid, 43–45
  acetone, 43–45
  diacetic acid, 43–45
  Gerhardt's test for, 47–48
  Hart's test for, 48
  β-hydroxybutyric acid, 43–45
  reagent test-strips for, 45–46
  Rothera's test for, 46–47
Ketonemia, 44
Ketonuria, 44
Ketosis, 44
Kidney, 2–7, *4*
Krebs cycle, 43

Lactose, 37
Leucine crystals, 84t, 94, *86, 94*
Leukocytes, 77–79, *77–79. See also* White
  blood cells
Lignin test, 97, 244
Lipuria, 120
Liver disease
  bilirubinuria in, 55–57
  leucine in, 94
  tyrosine crystals in, 96
Loop of Henle, 3–6, *4*
Lowe's syndrome, 253t, 256
Lycopodium, 122

Magnification, 72–73
Maltese-cross formation

fat, 115, 120, *122*
starch, 122, *123, 227*
Maltose, 37
Mannose, 37
Maple syrup urine disease, 13, 253t, 255t, 256
  leucine in, 94
Maroteaux-Lamy syndrome, 255
Melanin, 12, 246–247
  bromine test for, 246–247
  ferric chloride test for, 246
Melanogen, 12, 246
  Thormählen test for, 247
Melanoma, malignant, 246
  urine color in, 12
Metabolism, inborn errors of, 250–259
  Acetest for, 258
  aminoaciduria as, 251–252
  cetyltrimethylammonium bromide test for, 255–256
  cyanide–nitroprusside test for, 257–258
  dinitrophenylhydrazine test for, 256–257
  ferric chloride test for, 254, 255t
  manifestations of, 251
  ninhydrin test of, 259
  nitrosonaphthol test for, 258–259
  screening tests for, 252–259, 253t
Methyl red, 26
Methylene blue, 12
Microhematuria, 49
Microscope
  brightfield, 71
  colored filter technique for, 71
  focus of, 72, *73*
  interference contrast, 70–71
  magnification of, 72–73
  phase contrast, 70–71
  polarized light technique in, 71
  subdued light for, 72
  use of, 72–74, *73*
Microscopic examination, 69–132
  artifacts in, 122–129
  casts in, 107–116
  cells in, 74–81
  crystals in, 83–107
  miscellaneous structures in, 116–120
  parasites in, 129–132
Midstream specimen, 7–8
Mixed cast, *197, 211, 213, 215*
Modified Ehrlich's reagent, 262
Morquio's syndrome, 255

Mucopolysaccharides, increased, 255
Mucous, *175, 181, 195, 219*
Mucous threads, 118–120, *119*
Multiple myeloma, 34
Myocardial infarction, 52
Myoglobinuria, 12, 52–55
  ammonium sulfate test for, 55

Nephritis, 7, 49
Nephron, 2–6, *4*
Nephrosis, 7
Ninhydrin test, 253t, 259
Nitrite test, 64–65
Nitrosonaphthol test, 253t, 258–259
N-Multistix, 22
N-Multistix SG, 18

Oasthouse disease, 256
  leucine in, 94
  tyrosine crystals in, 96
Ochronosis, 245
Odor of urine, 13
Oil droplets, 125, *126*
Oil Red O stain, 70
Oliguria, 6
Osmolality
  freezing point in, 19
  specific gravity vs, 18–19
  vapor pressure depression in, 19
Osmometer, 19

Parasites, 129–132
  Enterobius vermicularis, 129, *131*
  Schistosoma haematobium, 132, *132*
  Trichomonas vaginalis, 129, *131*
Pass-through phenomenon, 41
Pentoses, 37
Peritubular capillaries, 4
pH of urine, 23–26
  bromthymol blue and, 26
  methyl red and, 26
  reagent test-strips for, 26
  regulation of, 25–26
Phenazopyridine, 12

Phenistix
  inborn errors of metabolism, 254
  phenylketonuria and, 249–250, 249t
Phenothiazine, 249, 249t
Phenylalanine metabolism, 245, *245*
Phenylketonuria, 247–250, 256, *248*
  ferric chloride test for, 250
  Guthrie test for, 248–249
  Phenistix for, 249–250, 249t
Phenylpyruvic oligophrenia, 247
Phosphates, amorphous, 13, 72, 84t, 102–
      103, *73, 101, 103, 171, 173, 177, 179,*
      205, 237
Phosphate plate, *105, 177, 179, 205, 237*
Pinworm, 129, *131, 237, 239*
Poisoning, salicylate, 25, 249
Pollen granules, 125
Polydipsia, 36
Polyphagia, 36
Polyuria, 6, 36
Porphobilinogen, 62, 63, 259–264
  Hoesch test for, 264
  Watson-Schwartz test for, 262–264
Porphyrin, 259–264, 260t, *260*
  precursors of, 260t
  screening test for, 261–262
Porphyrinuria, 12
Preservatives for urine, 8–9
Protein, 26–35
  Bence-Jones, 33–35. *See also* Bence-Jones
      protein
  Tamm-Horsfall, 27, 107, 108, 111
Protein error of indicators principle, 29
Proteinuria
  absence of, 28
  benign, 28
  heat and acetic acid test for, 32
  Heller's ring test for, 32–33
  glomerular, 27
  minimal, 28
  moderate, 27
  orthostatic or postural, 28
  reagent test-strips for, 29–31
  Robert's ring test for, 33
  screening tests for, 29–35
  severe, 27
  sulfosalicylic acid and, 31
  tubular, 27
Proximal convoluted tubule, 3–5
Prussian blue reaction, 243
Pyelonephritis, 7

Pyridium, 12
Pyuria, 78–79

Quality control, 65–67

Radiographic dye crystals, 84t, 98, *98–100,*
      167–169
Reagent strips
  bilirubin and, 59–60
  description of, 22–23
  glycosuria and, 38–40, 38t
  ketones and, 45–46
  leukocyte, 243–244
  occult blood and, 53–54
  pH, 26
  procedure for, 23
  protein and, 29–31
  specific gravity, 18
  types of, 24t
  urobilinogen and, 62–63
Red blood cells, 49–50, 74–77, *75–76, 135,*
      137, 185, 187, 189, 191, 195, 197, 201,
      217, 219
  bilirubin-stained, *213*
  differentiation of, 74–75, *76*
  focus change with, 75, *76*
  normal presence of, 76
  reporting number of, 74
  yeast cells vs, 75–76
Red cell casts, 108–109, *111, 191, 193, 215*
  convoluted, *191*
  degenerating, *193*
Reducing substances, 36–43, 253t, 254
  Benedict's qualitative test for, 42–43
  Clinitest for, 40–42
  copper reduction test for, 40–43
  fructose as, 37
  galactose as, 37
  lactose as, 37
  maltose as, 37
  mannose as, 37
  pentoses as, 37
  screening for, 40–43
Refractive index, 16
Refractometer, 16–18, *17*
Rejection, allograft, 111
Renal failure casts, 108

Renal tubular acidosis, 25
Renal tubular epithelial cells, 80, *80, 135, 139*
Renografin crystals, 98, *99*
Reticuloendothelial system, 55
Robert's ring test, 33
Rothera's test, 46–47
Rous test, 243
Run-over, 26

Salicylate poisoning, 25
    Phenistix for, 249
Sanfilippo syndrome, 255
Scheie's syndrome, 255
Schistosoma haematobium, 132, *132*
Sediment, urinary
    atlas of, 133–239
    preparation of, 72–74
Shadow cells, 74
Skatole, 62
Smith iodine test, 61
Sodium cyanide-sodium nitroprusside test,
    92, 253t, 257–258
Sodium urate crystals, 84t, 90–92, *86, 92,*
    155, 157
Solubility characteristics of crystals, 84t
Special screening procedures, 241–264
Specific gravity, 13–19, *15, 17*
    falling drop method for, 67
    hypersthenuria and, 14
    hyposthenuria and, 14
    increased vs decreased, 14–15
    isosthenuria and, 14
    normal range of, 14
    osmolality vs, 18–19
    protein and glucose correction in, 14
    reagent strips for, 18
    refractometer for, 16–18, *17*
    urinometer for, 15–16, *15*
Spermatozoa, 118, *119, 219*
Squamous epithelial cells, 81, *82, 135, 137,*
    139, 141, 153, 161, 163, 183, 195, 237
    sheet of, *141*
Starch crystals, 122, *123, 225, 227*
    Maltese-cross formation in, *227*
Sternheimer-Malbin supravital stain, 70
Stix, 242–243
Stones (calculi), 83
Sudan III stain, 70
Sudan IV stain, 70

Sulfonamide crystals, 97, 244, *97*
Sulfosalicylic acid, 31
Suprapubic aspiration, 7

Talcum powder, 125, *128, 237*
Tamm-Horsfall protein, 27, 107, 108, 111
Thormählen test, 247
Threshold substances, 5
Thymol, 9
Timed specimen collection, 9
Tobacco smoking, 50
Toluene, 8
Toluene sulfonic acid test, 35
Transitional epithelial cells, 81, *81–82, 135,*
    141
Trauma, 49–50
Trichomonas vaginalis, 129, *131*
Triple phosphate crystals, 84t, 102, *101, 102,*
    171–177
    calcium oxalate vs, *177*
    six-sided, *171*
Tubular degeneration, 111
Tubular necrosis, 111
Tubules, *4*
    collecting, 3, 6, *4*
    distal convoluted, 3, 5–6, *4*
    loop of Henle, 3, 5–6, *4*
    proximal convoluted, 3–6, *4*
Tyrosine crystals, 94–96, *86, 95, 165, 167*
Tyrosine metabolism, 245, 258, *245*
Tyrosinosis, 256, 258
    tyrosine crystals in, 96

Ultrafiltrate, 4
Urates, amorphous, 13, 84t, 90, *85, 91, 143,*
    153, 155, 193, 207, 221, 225, 235
    clumped, *143*
Urethra, 2, *3*
Uric acid crystals, 83, 84t, *85, 86–88, 143–*
    151
    atypical, *147*
    kidney stone and, *145*
    polarized, *88, 149, 151*
    pseudocast formation of, *151*
    rosette formation of, *145, 147, 149*
Urine
    appearance of, 13

Urine, (*continued*)
collection of, 7–9
color of, 10–13, 11t
constituents of, 6
formation of, 2–7
normal volume of, 6
odor of, 13
preservation of, 8–9
specific gravity of, 13–19, 67, *15, 17*
timed collection of, 9
Urinometer, 15–16, *15*
Urobilin, 10, 55, 62
Urobilinogen, 55–63
Ehrlich's qualitative test for, 63
normal pathway of, *56*
normal range for, 62
peak excretion of, 62
reagent test-strips for, 62–63
screening tests for, 61–63
timed specimens and, 9, 62
Watson-Schwartz test for, 262–264
Urochrome, 10
Uroerythrin, 10, 12
Urotron, 66–67

Vasa recta, 5
Vitamin C
bilirubin reagent test-strips, 59
calcium oxalate crystals and, 89
Clinitest and, 41
C-Stix and Stix for, 242–243
glucose oxidase test and, 39

leukocyte reagent test-strips, 244
nitrite test and, 65
occult blood reagent test-strips, 53–54

Watson-Schwartz test, 262–264
Waxy casts, 111–115, *115, 207–211*
bilirubin-stained, *207*
convoluted, *209, 211*
fiber vs, *231*
long, *209*
White blood cells, 77–79, *77–79, 135, 137,
139, 141, 157, 159, 161, 181, 185, 189,
195, 197, 199, 201, 203, 209, 213, 217,
223, 229, 237, 239*
bilirubin-stained, *139, 169, 207, 213*
Chemstrip L and Chemstrip 9 for, 243–244
clumped, 79, *78, 137*
differentiation of, 74–75, *76*
distorted, *137*
reagent test-strip for, 243–244
reporting number of, 74
swollen, *135*
White cell casts, 109–111, *111, 145, 189, 195–
199*
bilirubin-stained, *197*

X-ray dye crystals, 84t, 98, *98–100, 167, 169*

Yeast cells, 117, *117, 213, 217, 219*
red blood cells vs, 75–76
Yellow atrophy of liver, 94